Coronary Artery Bypass Grafting

Edited by Takashi Murashita

Published in London, United Kingdom

Coronary Artery Bypass Grafting
http://dx.doi.org/10.5772/intechopen.98027
Edited by Takashi Murashita

Contributors
Ahmad Farouk Musa, Artur Mikuliak, Vladlen Bazylev, Dmitry Tungusov, James Blankenship, Reed M. Otten, Murali P. Prabhakaran Vettath, Arunachalam Vellachamy Kannan, Gangadharan Nitin, Siddegowda Nagaraju Gururkirana, A.K. Baburajan, Raman Gopalakrishnan, Koroth Smera, Sridhar Kasturi, Thang Nguyen, An Viet Tran, Diem T. Nguyen, Son K. Tran, Trang H. Vo, Kien T. Nguyen, Phuong M. Nguyen, Suol T. Pham, Chu X. Duong, Bao L.T. Tran, Lien N.T. Tran, Han G. Diep, Minh V. Huynh, Thao H. Nguyen, Katja Taxis, Khanh D. Dang, Samuel Jacob, Pankaj Garg, Games Gramm, Saqib Masroor, Chuan Wang, Cheng Luo, BaoShi Zheng, Xiaoyong Xie

First published in London, United Kingdom, 2022 by IntechOpen
IntechOpen is the global imprint of INTECHOPEN LIMITED, registered in England and Wales, registration number: 11086078, 5 Princes Gate Court, London, SW7 2QJ, United Kingdom

British Library Cataloguing-in-Publication Data
A catalogue record for this book is available from the British Library

Additional hard and PDF copies can be obtained from orders@intechopen.com

Coronary Artery Bypass Grafting
Edited by Takashi Murashita
p. cm.
Print ISBN 978-1-80355-888-2
Online ISBN 978-1-80355-889-9
eBook (PDF) ISBN 978-1-80355-890-5

Meet the editor

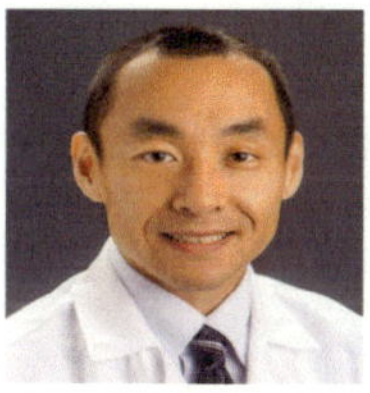

Takashi Murashita, MD, is an assistant professor in the Department of Surgery at the University of Missouri, Columbia, MO, USA. Dr. Murashita received his MD from Kyoto University Medical School, in Japan. His main interest is cardiac surgery, and he is a member of the Society of Thoracic Surgery, Eastern Cardiothoracic Surgical Society, and Asian Society for Cardiovascular and Thoracic Surgery. He has published 53 papers in peer-reviewed journals and 10 book chapters in open-access journals. He has been a member of editorial boards for 2 medical journals, and a member of ad-hoc manuscript reviewers for 16 medical journals.

Contents

Preface

The book, *Coronary Artery Bypass Grafting*, is an excellent update for health care professionals, taking care of patients who are suffering from severe coronary artery disease. The 8 chapters in this book were written by experts in their topics.

The first section described perioperative management for coronary artery disease. Chapter 1 discussed the most recent evidence of drug-related problems in coronary artery disease. Chapter 2 described the techniques of cardiac catheterization after CABG. Chapter 3 gave us an excellent review of the perioperative management of diabetic patients.

The second section described the various techniques of CABG. Chapter 4 described the most recent technique for off-pump CABG. Chapter 5 reported a unique technique of coronary-coronary bypass grafting. Chapter 6 discussed the role of CABG as a salvage procedure.

The last section discussed the comparison of CABG and percutaneous coronary intervention. Chapter 7 focused on the superiority of CABG vs PCI in diabetic patients. Chapter 8 discussed the superiority of CABG vs PCI in left main disease.

In conclusion, I believe this book will give us, health care professionals, the most updated information in the field of coronary artery bypass grafting.

Takashi Murashita, MD
Assistant Professor,
Division of Cardiothoracic Surgery,
University of Missouri,
Columbia, MO, USA

Section 1

Diagnosis and Management of Coronary Artery Disease

Chapter 1

Drug-Related Problems in Coronary Artery Diseases

An V. Tran, Diem T. Nguyen, Son K. Tran, Trang H. Vo, Kien T. Nguyen, Phuong M. Nguyen, Suol T. Pham, Chu X. Duong, Bao L.T. Tran, Lien N.T. Tran, Han G. Diep, Minh V. Huynh, Thao H. Nguyen, Katja Taxis, Khanh D. Dang and Thang Nguyen

Abstract

Coronary artery disease (CAD) remains the leading cause of mortality among cardiovascular diseases, responsible for 16% of the world's total deaths. According to a statistical report published in 2020, the global prevalence of CAD was estimated at 1655 per 100,000 people and is predicted to exceed 1845 by 2030. Annually, in the United States, CAD accounts for approximately 610,000 deaths and costs more than 200 billion dollars for healthcare services. Most patients with CAD need to be treated over long periods with a combination of drugs. Therefore, the inappropriate use of drugs, or drug-related problems (DRPs), can lead to many consequences that affect these patients' health, including decreased quality of life, increased hospitalization rates, prolonged hospital stays, increased overall health care costs, and even increased risk of morbidity and mortality. DRPs are common in CAD patients, with a prevalence of over 60%. DRPs must therefore be noticed and recognized by healthcare professionals. This chapter describes common types and determinants of DRPs in CAD patients and recommends interventions to limit their prevalence.

Keywords: cardiovascular diseases, ischemic heart disease, coronary artery disease, drug-related problems, interventions

1. Introduction

Worldwide, cardiovascular diseases (CVDs) are leading morbidity and mortality burdens. It has been estimated that 17.9 million people die from CVDs each year, representing 32% of all global deaths. The World Health Organization (WHO) defines CVDs as a group of disorders that include coronary artery disease (CAD), cerebrovascular disease, peripheral arterial disease, rheumatic heart disease, congenital heart disease, deep vein thrombosis, and pulmonary embolisms [1]. The world's biggest killer of all is ischemic heart disease, or CAD, responsible for 16% of the world's total deaths [2]. According to a statistical report published in 2020, the global prevalence of CAD was estimated at 1655 per 100,000 people and is predicted to exceed 1845 by 2030 [3]. In the United States, CAD accounts annually for approximately 610,000 deaths and costs more than 200 billion dollars for healthcare [4].

As most CAD patients are elderly and have multiple comorbidities, they need to use medication combinations over long periods, either for treatment or prophylaxis [5, 6]. One of the major strategies used for preventing CAD is antiplatelet therapy, and the most widely used antiplatelet agent tested is aspirin [6]. However, the therapeutic window of CAD drugs is very small, and inappropriate use can lead to many consequences that affect patients' health. For instance, aspirin plays a role in reducing the risk of cardiovascular events, but it also increases the risk of bleeding, the most common risk being gastrointestinal bleeding [7, 8]. Therefore, despite the benefit of the drug, it also causes problems that adversely affect health. Old age, polypharmacy, and comorbidities are significant risk factors for developing drug-related problems (DRPs) [9, 10].

A drug-related problem (DRP) has been defined as "an event or circumstance involving drug therapy that actually or potentially interferes with desired health outcomes" [11]. DRPs can have many negative consequences for patients and society, such as decreased quality of life for patients, increased hospitalization rates, prolonged hospital stays, increased overall healthcare costs, and even increased risk of morbidity and mortality [12–14]. For example, warfarin and oral antiplatelet agents have been reported to be implicated in nearly 50% of emergency hospital admissions of elderly Americans [15].

A further serious consequence of DRPs is the economic burden. DRPs accounted for a waste of $528.4 billion, equivalent to 16% of total US healthcare expenditures [16]. In studies of CVDs, the prevalence of patients with at least one DRP varied from nearly 30% to more than 90% [17–19]. A systematic review of DRPs concluded that the drugs most commonly involved were cardiovascular drugs [12]. In CAD patients, the drugs most implicated in DRPs were beta-blockers (BBs) (34.4%), followed by angiotensin-converting enzyme inhibitors (ACEI) (24.8%), statins (16.5%), and antithrombotics (13.1%) [20]. Different drugs are often associated with several different common DRPs. To illustrate, BBs were frequently involved in ineffective drug therapy, too low dosage, and the need for additional drug therapy, while ACEIs were commonly associated with too low dosage [20]. Studies in Ethiopia, Vietnam, and Spain have estimated that the mean numbers of DRPs for each patient with CAD were about 0.75, 0.92, and 1.51, respectively [17, 18, 21]. The prevalence of CAD patients with at least one DRP was 61.1% [21]. These statistics are relatively high and represent an alarming frequency of DRPs in patients with CAD. DRPs must therefore be noticed and recognized by healthcare professionals.

This chapter separates DRPs in CAD patients into 5 common subtypes: drug selection, dose selection, adverse drug-drug interactions (DDI), patient adherence, and cost issues. We also discuss determinants that increase the ratio of DRPs, and list interventions to limit their prevalence. Our goal is to provide health care providers with an overview of the extent of DRPs and their common types; these must be considered to ensure the safety and effectiveness of drug therapy.

2. Drug-related problems

2.1 Drug selection

Inappropriate drug selection is a common type of DRP in patients with CAD; it mainly includes ineffective drug therapy, a need for additional drug therapy, and prescription of drugs with contraindications. In an Ethiopian study, O.A. Abdela et al. found that, globally, the most common category of DRPs was inappropriate drug selection for CVDs (36.1%), and in particular for CAD (46.6%) [17]. Studies in Spain and Vietnam showed the prevalence of inappropriate drug selection of 19.4% and 3.5% for CAD patients [18, 21]. Inappropriate drug selection can have several causes. A study in Indonesia found that clinicians' critical factor influencing statin prescribing was their lack of awareness of specific details in current guideline recommendations. Although clinicians generally know the guidelines, they remain uncertain about how to determine the level of total cholesterol in combination with other cardiovascular risk factors like diabetes and hypertension [22].

Ineffective drug therapy occurs when the drug product used is not effective for the treatment of the medical condition [23]. A need for additional drug therapy exists when the medical condition requires additional drugs to achieve synergistic or additive effects [23]. A study by A.W. Tsige et al. in Ethiopia showed that among DRPs, the prevalence of need for additional drug therapy was 30.53%, and ineffective drug therapy was 26.9% [24]. In the Netherlands, J. Tra et al. conducted a study of prescriptions for patients discharged after CADs. They found that the angiotensin-converting enzyme inhibitor, one of the most important drugs in the prescribing guideline, was often missing (21.2%) [25]. In patients who have had acute coronary syndromes, it is vital to follow prescribing guidelines for secondary prevention to avoid further serious cardiovascular events. For example, according to a study on the prescription of secondary preventative cardiovascular therapies for non-ST elevation myocardial infarction (NSTEMI), adenosine-diphosphate receptor antagonist prescribing rates had significantly increased (76%) [26]. On the other hand, a study evaluating patient adherence to prescription guidelines after acute coronary syndrome indicated that adherence to lipid-lowering therapy was the lowest. The percentage of adherence to the criterion: 'Patient regardless of lipid level is prescribed a high-intensity statin either atorvastatin 40–80 mg or rosuvastatin 20–40 mg', was only 16.7% in the post-ST elevation myocardial infarction group, and 33.3% in the post-non-ST elevation acute coronary syndrome group [27]. A Canadian study found that only 61% of patients with stable coronary artery disease received optimal drug therapy involving concurrent use of β-blockers, ACE inhibitor/angiotensin receptor blockers, and statins [28]. Failure to prescribe drugs that should be indicated for treatment or prevention reduces the effectiveness of treatment. For example, after myocardial infarction, patients who have conditions like heart failure, pulmonary disease, and older age are often prescribed beta-blockade therapy, which is ineffective. However, patients without these conditions benefit from such therapy [29]. Ineffective drug therapy and a need for additional drugs can lead to increased medical costs, potential drug interactions, and decreased patient adherence [30].

Medicines that cause harm to the patient or negative interaction with a combination drug are called contraindicated medicines [31]. In a multicenter study in France, research on physicians' acceptance of pharmacists' daily routine interventions revealed that contraindication was the most identified DRP (21.3%) [32]. However, studies on CAD patients in Vietnam and Ethiopia showed that the prevalence of contraindicated medicines leading to DRPs was only approximately 0% and 2%, respectively [17, 21]. Therefore, in the latter two countries, among CAD patients, this issue is less common than in other DRPs.

Increasing the role of clinical pharmacists and the application of prescription management software in the prescribing process to check contraindication and interaction could be effective interventions to minimize such problems. For patients to be treated with appropriate drugs, clinicians should follow treatment guidelines and update their recommendations. In addition, the patient's response to treatment should be monitored by clinical examination and tests, and if necessary, a change of drug to suit the patient's condition.

2.2 Dose selection

Inappropriate dose selection includes both too high and too low [23]. A study in Spain by P. Gastelurrutia et al. found that inappropriate dose selection was one of the most frequently identified DRPs, with a prevalence of 22% [33], and a study in Turkey by Urbina, Olatz et al. found inappropriate dose selection in CAD patients to have a prevalence of 41% [18]. In a Vietnamese study by T.T.A. Truong et al., this prevalence was 22.2% [21]. Inappropriate dose selection can take place for several reasons. For example, ignoring comorbidities that affect the pharmacodynamics of a drug, such as hepatic or renal failure, can lead to inappropriate dose selection. Patients with renal and hepatic dysfunction require lower doses; otherwise, failure of excretion or breakdown of the drug can cause toxicity [34]. Furthermore, differing characteristics of patients, such as weight and body mass index, can make a prescribed dose too low or high for the patient's needs.

Sometimes high dosage prescription was considered when the duration of drug therapy was regarded as too long, possibly leading to unwanted side-effects for the patient [23]. In Spain and Vietnam, patients with CAD had a prevalence of high dose prescriptions of 8.6% and 0.1%, respectively [18, 21]. A study by Simon B. Dimmitt et al. had found that statin doses around an estimated effective dose of 50 (ED50) could reduce myocardial infarction (25%) and mortality (10%). However, the high dosage can also increase adverse events: myopathy was shown to increase 29-fold, and liver dysfunction as much as 9-fold [35]. A national study in America reported that overdoses led to nearly two-thirds of emergency hospitalizations [15]. Because the therapeutic window of CVD drugs in general, and CAD drugs in particular, is very small, an overdose is very severe and can lead to death. For example, an indirect sympathomimetic overdose can result in tachycardia, hypertension, stroke, and acute myocardial infarction [36]. Furthermore, in patients with renal dysfunction or renal failure, drugs that are eliminated by the kidney should be dosed proportionally according to creatinine clearance [37].

In contrast, a too low dosage means that the dose is not sufficient to produce the desired response [23]. In Spain and Vietnam, DRPs of patients with CAD occurring due to low dosage prescriptions were 7.9% and 22.1%, respectively [18, 21]. Taking too low a dose fails to achieve the desired therapeutic goal, increasing the possibility of cardiovascular events [23]. A systematic overview of randomized trial studies in patients with risk of cardiovascular disease found that a dose of aspirin between 75 and 150 mg daily gives adequate prophylaxis; doses lower than 75 mg daily are less effective [38]. A study was conducted in patients with acute coronary syndrome after stent implantation to compare the efficacy of different doses of rosuvastatin [39]. This study concluded that high doses of rosuvastatin could postpone ventricular remodeling, decrease the prevalence of adverse events, and significantly improve long-term prognosis.

To limit problems related to dose selection, doctors need to pay attention to each patient's condition, comorbidities, and characteristics affecting drug pharmacokinetics and monitor and adjust drug dose depending on the tolerance of the individual patient. In addition, the clinical pharmacist can help to calculate the appropriate drug dose for each patient. Furthermore, the application software should be developed to assist in dose calculation for special populations like elderly patients or liver and/or kidney disease patients.

2.3 Adverse drug-drug interaction

Adverse drug-drug interactions (DDIs) occur when drug interaction leads to undesirable reactions that are not dose-related [23]. In patients with heart failure in Ethiopia, DDIs were the most common cause of DRPs, with a prevalence of 27.3% in 2020 and 33.4% in 2021 [24, 40]. However, a study in Taiwan found DDIs to be the second most common DRP (29.6%) [41]. In patients with CAD in Ethiopia and Vietnam, DDIs had prevalences of 21.2% and 19.3%, respectively [21, 40]. Often, patients with CAD have to take multiple medications for a long time [5], and other drugs must frequently be used to treat co-morbidities. However, the greater the number of drugs, the greater the risk of drug-drug interactions [5].

The most common DDI found in patients with heart failure was the combined use of spironolactone and digoxin, possibly resulting in increased digoxin toxicity [40]. A systematic review of secondary prevention of adverse ischemic events found that a regimen including aspirin plus clopidogrel led to a significantly higher rate of hemorrhagic events than other regimens (aspirin alone, plus ticlopidine or cilostazol, etc.) [6]. Another common drug-drug interaction between clopidogrel and proton pump inhibitors (PPIs) in patients with CAD. Clopidogrel is a P2Y12 receptor inhibitor and one of the two components of dual antiplatelet therapy [42]. PPIs are recommended for patients on dual antiplatelet therapy with a history or high risk of gastrointestinal bleeding [43]. Adverse drug interactions reduce the effectiveness of treatment. For example, some PPIs, such as omeprazole and esomeprazole, reduce the antiplatelet effect of clopidogrel by inhibiting the CYP2C19-mediated conversion of clopidogrel to the active metabolite in the liver [44]. In addition, concomitant clopidogrel-PPI therapy appears to increase the risk of major adverse cardiovascular events [45]. Meanwhile, PPIs such as lansoprazole and dexlansoprazole have been found to have less effect, and pantoprazole and rabeprazole do not affect the metabolism of clopidogrel [46, 47]. Therefore, one of the four PPIs: pantoprazole, rabeprazole, lansoprazole, or dexlansoprazole, should be chosen, and omeprazole and esomeprazole should be avoided in patients requiring a combination of clopidogrel and PPI.

To limit adverse drug-drug interactions, clinicians can use drug interaction testing tools with the assistance of a clinical pharmacist. If a severe drug-drug interaction occurs, an alternative drug should be considered. Furthermore, an online drug interaction checker (Drug.com, Medscape, etc.) should be used for checking before prescribing to patients.

2.4 Patient nonadherence

Poor patient adherence is another common DRP in coronary artery disease. Nonadherence involves the failure of a patient to take medications appropriately due to personal factors [23]. Several studies have indicated that roughly 20% and more than 50% of CAD patients are non-adherent to prescribed medications [48–50]. Many factors can affect patient adherence to treatment: lack of motivation, failure to understand instructions, forgetfulness, the complexity of the regimen, polypharmacy, multiple daily doses, adverse side effects, high cost, failure to initiate treatment before discharge, and the physician's lack of knowledge of clinical indicators for the use of medications [51, 52]. In addition, older people have many unique difficulties that contribute to poor adherence [52], one of the main factors being forgetfulness [53]. Some studies indicate that long-term therapy involving CAD prophylaxis may decrease adherence. A Swedish study reported that the adherence rate in CAD patients after discharge rapidly decreased within 2 years. Statin, aspirin, and clopidogrel adherence rates decreased from 91.7% to 56.1%, 93.2% to 61.5%, and 81.9% to 39.4% respectively, 2 years after discharge [54].

Patient adherence greatly contributes to the success of treatment and secondary prevention strategies in CAD patients. Good adherence to evidence-based medication regimens, including β-blockers, angiotensin-converting enzyme inhibitors/angiotensin receptor blockers, antiplatelet drugs, and statins, has been shown to be associated with decreased risk of all-cause mortality (risk ratio 0.56; 95% confidence interval: 0.45–0.69), cardiovascular mortality (risk ratio 0.66; 95% confidence interval: 0.51–0.87), and cardiovascular hospitalization/myocardial infarction (risk ratio 0.61; 95% confidence interval: 0.45–0.82) [55]. In contrast, poor adherence can lead to major cardiovascular events, including death [56]. In Turkey, during one-year follow-up treatment, patients with acute coronary syndrome were found to have low adherence to statin therapy (17.8%) [57]. According to a study by C.A. Jackevicius et al. in the Canadian population, patients who did not use all of their discharge medications after acute coronary syndrome had an increased risk of death at 1 year [56]. The death rates among high-adherence and low-adherence were respectively 2310/14,345 (16%), and 261/1071 (24%) (adjusted hazard ratio, 1.25; 95% confidence interval, 1.09–1.42; $p = 0.001$). The study also found a similar but less pronounced dose-response-type adherence-mortality association for beta-blockers [58]. However, the harmful consequence of nonadherence depends on the type of medication. For example, the mortality rate was not associated with adherence to calcium channel blockers [58]. However, patients must adhere to the prescribed regimens to achieve treatment goals.

Drug counseling upon discharge and post-discharge follow-up may increase adherence [56]. When patients know their medical condition and the benefits of prescription medications, they are more motivated to take them exactly as recommended [59]. Moreover, appropriate prescribing upon discharge should be encouraged to improve patient adherence [52]. Prescribing fixed-dose combination pills instead of using multiple single drugs also helps to enhance adherence [60, 61]. A systematic review in low- and middle-income countries demonstrated considerable variation in nonadherence to antihypertensive medication [62]. Due to the overload of healthcare systems, especially in these low- and middle-income countries and during the COVID-19 pandemic, clinicians have too little time to educate patients [63]. A systematic review of 67 countries found that about half of the world's population spends 5 min or less with their primary care physicians [64]. Therefore, more attention should be paid to the role of the clinical pharmacist. Clinical pharmacists can help patients understand the benefits of each medication they take, the timing and frequency of administration, and signs of side effects; they can also encourage and monitor patient adherence. A systematic review of medication adherence interventions showed significant reductions in mortality risk among heart failure patients (relative risk, 0.89; 95% CI, 0.81, 0.99). A bulk of these interventions utilized medication education (s = 50) and disease education (s = 48) [65].

2.5 Cost issue

Medical costs for CAD have increased dramatically in recent years and are expected to rise even more [66]. The result is an increased economic burden for patients themselves and countries. For example, hospital admission for acute myocardial infarction requiring percutaneous coronary intervention costs an average of $20,000 [67]. In the USA, it has been calculated that in 2016 DRPs wasted $528.4 billion, equivalent to 16% of the total US healthcare expenditure for that year [16]. Furthermore, the cost of informal healthcare for CAD alone was estimated at $1 billion and projected to increase to $1.9 billion by 2035 [68]. According to M. Guerro-Prado et al., cost issues accounted for up to 6.5% of all DRPs. Unnecessary and unnecessarily expensive treatments were the main reasons for such problems [69]. Furthermore, cost issues are also related to physicians' prescriptions. A Chinese national study among 3362 primary healthcare sites showed that expensive medications were more likely to be prescribed than less costly alternatives, thus contributing to high medication costs [70]. Increased medication costs may likely reduce patient adherence and negatively affect their healthcare [51, 71]. Patients' discontinuation of medication therapies affects their treatment outcomes and increases the occurrence of adverse cardiovascular events [56]. To treat these events, the costs of treatment become even greater.

WHO has listed some interventions that may reduce costs. Such interventions include providing information; government communication is vital to raise public awareness of the importance of reducing cardiovascular risk factors. Further efforts to reduce medical costs include early disease detection, optimal treatment according to recommendations, and close patient management to limit complications, hospitalization, and death. Also recommended for patients with coronary artery disease are lifestyle changes that enhance the effectiveness of treatment, thereby reducing the number of drugs needed [72]. To further avoid adding to treatment costs, clinicians should avoid prescribing unnecessary extra drugs [70]. Finally, it is necessary to encourage individuals to participate in health insurance to reduce the financial burden of illness [72].

3. Conclusions

DRPs are a global problem, causing adverse consequences in cardiology in particular and medicine in general. Drug selection, dose selection, adverse drug-drug interactions, and patient adherence are the most common categories involved in DRPs. Inability to control DRPs can diminish healthcare outcomes and increase the prevalence of adverse cardiovascular events, and DRPs can also inhibit economic growth due to medication costs. To minimize the negative impacts of DRPs we propose several key solutions: (1) appropriate prescribing according to guidelines, (2) enhancing the role of clinical pharmacists in the identification and intervention of DRPs, and (3) developing tools to check for drug interactions and contraindications. More effective definition and recognition of DRPs and application of relevant interventions can help to limit these global problems.

Author details

An V. Tran[1], Diem T. Nguyen[1], Son K. Tran[1], Trang H. Vo[1], Kien T. Nguyen[1], Phuong M. Nguyen[1], Suol T. Pham[2], Chu X. Duong[2], Bao L.T. Tran[1], Lien N.T. Tran[1], Han G. Diep[2], Minh V. Huynh[3], Thao H. Nguyen[4], Katja Taxis[5], Khanh D. Dang[2]* and Thang Nguyen[2]*

1 Faculty of Medicine, Can Tho University of Medicine and Pharmacy, Can Tho, Vietnam

2 Department of Pharmacology and Clinical Pharmacy, Can Tho University of Medicine and Pharmacy, Can Tho, Vietnam

3 Department of Cardiology, Hue College of Medicine and Pharmacy, Hue University, Hue, Vietnam

4 Department of Clinical Pharmacy, University of Medicine and Pharmacy at Ho Chi Minh City, Ho Chi Minh City, Vietnam

5 Groningen Research Institute of Pharmacy, University of Groningen, Groningen, The Netherlands

*Address all correspondence to: ddkhanh@ctump.edu.vn and nthang@ctump.edu.vn

References

[1] World Health Organization, Cardiovascular diseases (CVDs). 2021. Available from: https://www.who.int/news-room/fact-sheets/detail/cardiovascular-diseases-(cvds) [Accessed: June 11, 2021]

[2] World Health Organization, The Top 10 Causes of Death. 2020. Available from: https://www.who.int/news-room/fact-sheets/detail/the-top-10-causes-of-death [Accessed: December 9, 2020]

[3] Khan MA et al. Global epidemiology of ischemic heart disease: Results from the Global Burden of Disease Study. Cureus. 2020;**12**(7):e9349

[4] Brown JC, Gerhardt TE, Kwon E. Risk factors for coronary artery disease. In: StatPearls. 2022, StatPearls Publishing Copyright ©. Treasure Island (FL): StatPearls Publishing LLC; 2022

[5] InformedHealth.org. Medication for the Long-Term Treatment of Coronary Artery Disease. 2006. Available from: https://www.ncbi.nlm.nih.gov/books/NBK355311/ [Accessed: July 27, 2017]

[6] Niu PP et al. Antiplatelet regimens in the long-term secondary prevention of transient ischaemic attack and ischaemic stroke: An updated network meta-analysis. BMJ Open. 2016;**6**(3):e009013

[7] Zhao B et al. Pros and cons of aspirin for the primary prevention of cardiovascular events: A secondary study of trial sequential analysis. Frontiers in Pharmacology. 2020;**11**:592116

[8] Weisman SM, Brunton S. Primary prevention of CVD with aspirin: Benefits vs risks. The Journal of Family Practice. 2021;**70**(6s):S41-s46

[9] Nivya K et al. Systemic review on drug related hospital admissions—A pubmed based search. Saudi Pharmaceutical Journal. 2015;**23**(1):1-8

[10] Al Hamid A et al. A systematic review of hospitalization resulting from medicine-related problems in adult patients. British Journal of Clinical Pharmacology. 2014;**78**(2):202-217

[11] Association. P.C.N.E. Pharmaceutical Care Network Europe Classification for Drug Related Problem V9.1. 2020. Available from: https://www.pcne.org/upload/files/417_PCNE_classification_V9-1_final.pdf

[12] Gayathri B et al. Drug related problems: A systemic literature review. International Journal of Clinical Pharmacology and Therapeutics. 2018;**9**(1):1409-1415

[13] Ayalew MB, Tegegn HG, Abdela OA. Drug related hospital admissions; a systematic review of the recent literatures. Bulletin of Emergency And Trauma. 2019;**7**(4):339-346

[14] Abraham RR. Drug related problems and reactive pharmacist interventions for inpatients receiving cardiovascular drugs. International Journal of Basic Medical Sciences and Pharmacy (IJBMSP). 2014;**3**(2):42-48

[15] Budnitz DS et al. Emergency hospitalizations for adverse drug events in older Americans. The New England Journal of Medicine. 2011;**365**(21):2002-2012

[16] Watanabe JH, McInnis T, Hirsch JD. Cost of prescription drug-related morbidity and mortality. The Annals of Pharmacotherapy. 2018;**52**(9):829-837

[17] Abdela OA et al. Risk factors for developing drug-related problems in

patients with cardiovascular diseases attending Gondar University Hospital, Ethiopia. Journal of Pharmacy and Bioallied Sciences. 2016;**8**(4):289-295

[18] Urbina O et al. Patient risk factors for developing a drug-related problem in a cardiology ward. Therapeutics and Clinical Risk Management. 2015;**11**:9-15

[19] Niquille A, Bugnon O. Relationship between drug-related problems and health outcomes: A cross-sectional study among cardiovascular patients. Pharmacy World & Science. 2010;**32**(4): 512-519

[20] Niriayo YL et al. Drug therapy problems and contributing factors in the management of heart failure patients in Jimma University Specialized Hospital, Southwest Ethiopia. PLoS One. 2018;**13**(10):e0206120

[21] Truong TTA et al. Drug-related problems in prescribing for coronary artery diseases in Vietnam: Cross-sectional study. Tropical Medicine & International Health. 2019;**24**(11):1335-1340

[22] Irawati S et al. Key factors influencing the prescribing of statins: A qualitative study among physicians working in primary healthcare facilities in Indonesia. BMJ Open. 2020;**10**(6):e035098

[23] Cipolle RJ et al. Pharmaceutical Care Practice: The Clinician's Guide: The Clinician's Guide. Americas New York City, United States: McGraw-Hill Medical; 2004

[24] Tsige AW, Yikna BB, Altaye BM. Drug-related problems among ambulatory heart failure patients on follow-up at Debre Berhan comprehensive specialized hospital, Ethiopia. Therapeutics and Clinical Risk Management. 2021;**17**:1165-1175

[25] Tra J et al. Adherence to guidelines for the prescription of secondary prevention medication at hospital discharge after acute coronary syndrome: A multicentre study. Netherlands Heart Journal. 2015;**23**(4):214-221

[26] Venkatason P et al. Trends and variations in the prescribing of secondary preventative cardiovascular therapies for non-ST elevation myocardial infarction (NSTEMI) in Malaysia. European Journal of Clinical Pharmacology. 2018;**74**(7):953-960

[27] Al-Taweel D, Awad A. Development and validation of medication assessment tools to evaluate prescribing adherence to evidence-based guidelines for secondary prevention of coronary heart disease in post-acute coronary syndromes patients in Kuwait. PLoS One. 2020;**15**(11):e02416 33-e0241633

[28] Chun S et al. Predictors and outcomes of routine versus optimal medical therapy in stable coronary heart disease. The American Journal of Cardiology. 2015;**116**(5):671-677

[29] Gottlieb SS, McCarter RJ, Vogel RA. Effect of beta-blockade on mortality among high-risk and low-risk patients after myocardial infarction. The New England Journal of Medicine. 1998;**339**(8):489-497

[30] By J. Mark Ruscin, S.A.L. Drug-Related Problems in Older Adults. 2021. Available from: https://www.msdmanuals.com/professional/geriatrics/drug-therapy-in-older-adults/drug-related-problems-in-older-adults

[31] Company, F.A.D. Contraindication. 2004. Available from: https://www.tabers.com/tabersonline/view/Tabers-Dictionary/754565/all/contraindication

[32] Bedouch P et al. Assessment of clinical pharmacists' interventions in French hospitals: Results of a multicenter study. The Annals of Pharmacotherapy. 2008;**42**(7):1095-1103

[33] Gastelurrutia P et al. Negative clinical outcomes associated with drug-related problems in heart failure (HF) outpatients: Impact of a pharmacist in a multidisciplinary HF clinic. Journal of Cardiac Failure. 2011;**17**(3):217-223

[34] Tariq RA et al. Medication Dispensing Errors and Prevention. In: StatPearls. Treasure Island (FL), United States: StatPearls Publishing; 2022

[35] Dimmitt SB, Stampfer HG, Warren JB. The pharmacodynamic and clinical trial evidence for statin dose. British Journal of Clinical Pharmacology. 2018;**84**(6):1128-1135

[36] Mladěnka P et al. Comprehensive review of cardiovascular toxicity of drugs and related agents. Medicinal Research Reviews. 2018;**38**(4):1332-1403

[37] Doogue MP, Polasek TM. Drug dosing in renal disease. Clinical Biochemist Reviews. 2011;**32**(2):69-73

[38] Antithrombotic Trialist's Collaboration. Collaborative meta-analysis of randomised trials of antiplatelet therapy for prevention of death, myocardial infarction, and stroke in high risk patients. BMJ. 2002;**324**(7329):71-86

[39] Guo J et al. Study on the effect of different doses of rosuvastatin on ventricular remodeling in patients with acute coronary syndrome after emergency percutaneous coronary intervention. European Review for Medical and Pharmacological Sciences. 2017;**21**(19):4457-4463

[40] Seid E et al. Evaluation of drug therapy problems, medication adherence and treatment satisfaction among heart failure patients on follow-up at a tertiary care hospital in Ethiopia. PLoS One. 2020;**15**(8):e0237781

[41] Hsu WT, Shen LJ, Lee CM. Drug-related problems vary with medication category and treatment duration in Taiwanese heart failure outpatients receiving case management. Journal of the Formosan Medical Association. 2016;**115**(5):335-342

[42] Ferri N, Corsini A, Bellosta S. Pharmacology of the new P2Y12 receptor inhibitors: Insights on pharmacokinetic and pharmacodynamic properties. Drugs. 2013;**73**(15):1681-1709

[43] Levine GN et al. 2016 ACC/AHA Guideline Focused Update on Duration of Dual Antiplatelet Therapy in Patients With Coronary Artery Disease: A Report of the American College of Cardiology/American Heart Association Task Force on Clinical Practice Guidelines: An Update of the 2011 ACCF/AHA/SCAI Guideline for Percutaneous Coronary Intervention, 2011 ACCF/AHA Guideline for Coronary Artery Bypass Graft Surgery, 2012 ACC/AHA/ACP/AATS/PCNA/SCAI/STS Guideline for the Diagnosis and Management of Patients With Stable Ischemic Heart Disease, 2013 ACCF/AHA Guideline for the Management of ST-Elevation Myocardial Infarction, 2014 AHA/ACC Guideline for the Management of Patients With Non–ST-Elevation Acute Coronary Syndromes, and 2014 ACC/AHA Guideline on Perioperative cardiovascular evaluation and management of patients undergoing noncardiac surgery. Circulation. 2016;**134**(10):e123-e155

[44] Norgard NB, Mathews KD, Wall GC. *Drug-drug interaction between clopidogrel and the proton pump inhibitors*. The Annals of Pharmacotherapy. 2009;**43**(7):1266-1274

[45] Serbin MA, Guzauskas GF, Veenstra DL. Clopidogrel-proton pump inhibitor drug-drug interaction and risk of adverse clinical outcomes among PCI-treated ACS patients: A meta-analysis. Journal of Managed Care & Specialty Pharmacy. 2016;**22**(8):939-947

[46] Frelinger AL 3rd et al. A randomized, 2-period, crossover design study to assess the effects of dexlansoprazole, lansoprazole, esomeprazole, and omeprazole on the steady-state pharmacokinetics and pharmacodynamics of clopidogrel in healthy volunteers. Journal of the American College of Cardiology. 2012;**59**(14):1304-1311

[47] Wang ZY et al. Pharmacokinetic drug interactions with clopidogrel: Updated review and risk management in combination therapy. Therapeutics and Clinical Risk Management. 2015;**11**:449-467

[48] Molloy GJ et al. Intentional and unintentional non-adherence to medications following an acute coronary syndrome: A longitudinal study. Journal of Psychosomatic Research. 2014;**76**(5):430-432

[49] Ali MA et al. Frequency and predictors of non-adherence to lifestyle modifications and medications after coronary artery bypass grafting: A cross-sectional study. Indian Heart Journal. 2017;**69**(4):469-473

[50] Padilha JC et al. Prevalence of pharmacological adherence in patients with coronary artery disease and associated factors. Revista Latino-Americana de Enfermagem. 2021;**29**:e3464

[51] Cheng K et al. Evidence of poor adherence to secondary prevention after acute coronary syndromes: Possible remedies through the application of new technologies. Open Heart. 2015;**2**(1):e000166

[52] Sengstock D et al. Under-prescribing and non-adherence to medications after coronary bypass surgery in older adults: Strategies to improve adherence. Drugs & Aging. 2012;**29**(2):93-103

[53] Bastani P et al. Determinants affecting medication adherence in the elderly: A qualitative study. Aging Medicine. 2021;**4**(1):35-41

[54] Glader EL et al. Persistent use of secondary preventive drugs declines rapidly during the first 2 years after stroke. Stroke. 2010;**41**(2):397-401

[55] Du L et al. The impact of medication adherence on clinical outcomes of coronary artery disease: A meta-analysis. European Journal of Preventive Cardiology. 2017;**24**(9):962-970

[56] Jackevicius CA, Li P, Tu JV. Prevalence, predictors, and outcomes of primary nonadherence after acute myocardial infarction. Circulation. 2008;**117**(8):1028-1036

[57] Şimşek B et al. In-hospital statin initiation characteristics and one-year statin adherence rates in patients hospitalised for acute coronary syndrome. Acta Cardiologica. 2021;**76**(8):852-858

[58] Rasmussen JN, Chong A, Alter DA. Relationship between adherence to evidence-based pharmacotherapy and long-term mortality after acute myocardial infarction. JAMA. 2007;**297**(2):177-186

[59] Jimmy B, Jose J. Patient medication adherence: Measures in daily practice. Oman Medical Journal. 2011;**26**(3):155-159

[60] Lauffenburger JC, Landon JE, Fischer MA. Effect of combination

therapy on adherence among US patients initiating therapy for hypertension: A cohort study. Journal of General Internal Medicine. 2017;**32**(6):619-625

[61] Yusuf S et al. Combination pharmacotherapy to prevent cardiovascular disease: Present status and challenges. European Heart Journal. 2014;**35**(6):353-364

[62] Nielsen J et al. Non-adherence to anti-hypertensive medication in low- and middle-income countries: A systematic review and meta-analysis of 92443 subjects. Journal of Human Hypertension. 2017;**31**(1):14-21

[63] Hamid H, Abid Z, Amir A, Rehman TU, Akram W, Mehboob T. Current burden on healthcare systems in low- and middle-income countries: Recommendations for emergency care of COVID-19 [published online ahead of print, 2020 Aug 9]. Drugs Ther Perspect. 2020:1-3. DOI: 10.1007/s40267-020-00766-2

[64] Irving G et al. International variations in primary care physician consultation time: A systematic review of 67 countries. BMJ Open. 2017;7(10):e017902

[65] Ruppar TM et al. Medication adherence interventions improve heart failure mortality and readmission rates: Systematic review and meta-analysis of controlled trials. Journal of the American Heart Association. 2016;**5**(6):1-18

[66] International, R. Cardiovascular Disease Costs Will Exceed $1 Trillion by 2035: Nearly Half of Americans Will Develop Pre-Existing Cardiovascular Disease Conditions, Analysis Shows. 2017. Available from: www.sciencedaily.com/releases/2017/02/170214162750.htm

[67] Cowper PA et al. Acute and 1-year hospitalization costs for acute myocardial infarction treated with percutaneous coronary intervention: Results from the TRANSLATE-ACS registry. Journal of the American Heart Association. 2019;**8**(8):e011322-e011322

[68] Dunbar SB et al. Projected costs of informal caregiving for cardiovascular disease: 2015 to 2035: A policy statement from the American Heart Association. Circulation. 2018;**137**(19):e558-e577

[69] Guerro-Prado M, Olmo-Revuelto MA, Catalá-Pindado M. Prevalence of medication-related problems in complex chronic patients and opportunities for improvement. Farmacia Hospitalaria. 2018;**42**(5):197-199

[70] Su M et al. Availability, cost, and prescription patterns of antihypertensive medications in primary health care in China: A nationwide cross-sectional survey. Lancet. 2017;**390**(10112):2559-2568

[71] McIntyre D et al. What are the economic consequences for households of illness and of paying for health care in low- and middle-income country contexts? Social Science & Medicine. 2006;**62**(4):858-865

[72] Essue BM et al. The effectiveness of interventions to reduce the household economic burden of illness and injury: A systematic review. Bulletin of the World Health Organization. 2015;**93**(2):102-12b

Chapter 2

Cardiac Catheterization after Bypass Surgery

Reed M. Otten and James Blankenship

Abstract

After coronary artery bypass graft (CABG) surgery, the typical patient will have progression of the original native coronary disease as well as atherosclerosis of the bypass grafts. When this leads to angina or myocardial infarction, repeat cardiac catheterization may be necessary. However, the risks of catheterization in post-CABG patients are higher than in non-CABG patients, and the benefits are smaller, so optimal medical therapy should be employed and clear indications should be present before post-CABG catheterization is undertaken. In the past decade, two advancements have been made in strategies for post-CABG catheterization. First, for patients with a left internal mammary artery graft, left radial access should be routinely used and is safer than femoral access. Second, diseased saphenous vein bypass grafts may offer a retrograde approach to chronic total occlusions of the native artery. When successful, retrograde stenting of the bypassed native coronary artery is more durable than interventions on the saphenous vein graft supplying it. This chapter summarizes indications, techniques, and tricks of catheterization and strategies for coronary intervention in patients with prior CABG.

Keywords: bypass graft surgery, saphenous vein graft, cardiac catheterization, vein graft stenting

1. Introduction

The two main methods of revascularization in coronary artery disease are percutaneous coronary intervention (PCI) and coronary artery bypass surgery (CABG). In modern medicine, coronary artery bypass surgery is mostly reserved for the most severe or complex coronary artery disease. Patients who are status post-CABG can develop further coronary disease and myocardial ischemia in the years following surgery. As in any other patient who is suspected of having coronary artery disease, cardiac catheterization provides the definitive test (angiography) and is often the treatment modality of choice (PCI) in patients with prior CABG. This chapter aims to highlight the most important aspects of cardiac catheterization, coronary angiography, bypass graft angiography, and percutaneous coronary intervention in patients who are status post coronary artery bypass surgery.

1.1 Types of bypass grafts

The left internal mammary artery (LIMA) graft to the left anterior descending (LAD) coronary artery provides CABG with its primary benefit over PCI in multi-vessel disease. The LIMA is a branch of the left subclavian artery, which itself branches from the aortic arch. The LIMA arises from the inferior-anterior aspect of the subclavian artery and courses caudally down the left chest. This graft is generally used as an in situ graft with its free end anastomosed to a coronary artery (usually the LAD).

Other than the LIMA, other bypass graft options include the right internal mammary artery (RIMA), radial artery, and saphenous veins. Most often grafts to arteries other than the LAD utilize saphenous veins. These are harvested from the legs and an anastomosis is created most often from the ascending aorta to the target coronary artery. Rarely an in situ gastroepiploic artery is anastomosed to the right coronary artery or the inferior epigastric artery is harvested and used as a free graft anastomosed to the aorta.

Free arterial grafts are superior to saphenous vein grafts (SVGs) [1, 2] however their use is limited by several factors. Radial artery grafts must meet stringent requirements before harvesting for use in CABG. Rarely radial arteries cannot be used because they are too small, previously traumatized (i.e. prior transradial catheterizations), or supply all blood flow to the hand. The RIMA can also be used, either in situ or as a free graft, but the use of both the LIMA and the RIMA is associated with an increased risk of sternal wound infections [2]. For these reasons, SVGs remain the most frequently used graft other than the LIMA.

1.2 Configurations of bypass grafts

Most commonly grafts have a single origin and single terminal anastomosis. However, several variations are used by surgeons:

- "Jump" or sequential grafts: Often a LIMA or SVG will be anastomosed side-to-side to an artery or branch and then the distal graft will be anastomosed end-to-side to a second artery or branch. For the LIMA it is typical to anastomose to a LAD-diagonal branch and terminate at the distal LAD. SVGs are often jumped from a first to a second obtuse marginal or from a right coronary artery (RCA) posterior descending branch to an RCA-posterolateral branch.

- "Snake" or long circular grafts: In a technique that has fallen out of favor but still may be found occasionally, a single long saphenous vein graft is anastomosed to the aorta and then anastomosed side-to-side to the LAD and/or branches then to the circumflex branches and finally anastomosed end-to-side to the RCA.

- Under unusual circumstances (e.g., a third CABG surgery) a surgeon may anastomose an SVG from the descending aorta to a coronary artery (usually the circumflex).

- An in situ RIMA may be anastomosed to the circumflex, right coronary artery, or the right coronary posterior descending branch.

- An in situ gastroepiploic artery may be anastomosed to the right coronary artery. This can be easily cannulated using a Judkins right (JR4) catheter to identify the hepato-splenic trunk, advancing the catheter over the wire into the hepatic artery and then the gastro-epiploic artery.

- Y grafts: Surgeons may anastomose a free radial artery to a LIMA with the radial graft going to a diagonal branch of the left anterior descending and the LIMA ending at the LAD. Rarely surgeons will anastomose a SVG segment to an SVG in a similar fashion.

- Common aortic "hoods" or "buttons". Occasionally surgeons will anastomose two SVGs to a single spot on the aorta so that both arise from the same point.

1.3 Natural history of bypass grafts

Arterial grafts are more durable than venous grafts. When grafted to the LAD, the LIMA graft has a five-year patency rate of 91%, whereas vein grafts had a five-year patency rate of 78% [3, 4]. In patients who underwent CABG between 1995 and 2010, at a 7-year follow-up the patency of the LIMA was 87%, the patency of a radial artery graft to the RCA or LCx was 82%, and the patency of saphenous vein grafts was 58% [5].

Three processes lead to SVG failure, and the mechanism of failure can be predicted by the timing of failure. A useful rule of thumb is that about 10% of grafts occlude in under 1 month due to thrombosis or surgical issues, about 10% occlude between 1 month and 1 year due to intimal proliferation, in about 2–3% more occlude per year due to accelerated atherosclerosis. Within the first month after CABG, thrombosis (i.e. due to hypercoagulability) and technical failure (i.e. damage to or defects of the graft) are the predominant mechanisms. From the first month to the first year after CABG intimal hyperplasia is the predominant mechanism, a process in which smooth muscle cells proliferate and fibroblasts lay down extracellular matrix (also known as "arterialization" of the graft) in response to exposure to arterial pressures. And beyond the first year of CABG atherosclerosis is the predominant mechanism, a process that is accelerated in SVGs as compared to native arteries and in which unstable plaques often form [6].

1.4 Indications for cardiac catheterization after CABG

The 2012 Appropriate Use Criteria for Diagnostic Catheterization provide indications for cardiac catheterization in patients with prior CABG [7]. Common indications include acute coronary syndromes or electrical instability. Emergent coronary angiography may be indicated for postoperative CABG patients who have clear signs of ischemia, unexplained hemodynamic instability, low cardiac output syndrome, electrical instability, diffuse electrocardiogram changes, new ischemic wall motion abnormalities, or very large troponin elevations after CABG. Troponin elevations of >10x the upper limits of normal qualify as type 5 myocardial infarction (MI) in the Fourth Universal Definition of Myocardial Infarction [6, 8, 9].

For stable patients, the indications are more limited. In general, asymptomatic patients should not undergo catheterization unless there is other evidence of extensive ischemia. Specifically, a small or even moderate-sized ischemic abnormality on stress testing would not warrant catheterization in a patient with no symptoms or atypical symptoms. The indication for catheterization strengthens as symptoms increase despite guideline-directed medical therapy or as the evidence for extensive ischemia increases. Consideration of catheterization in patients after CABG must balance the risks of catheterization (which are about twice those of diagnostic coronary arteriography in non-CABG patients) and the risks of subsequent PCI against the benefits of symptom relief or of diagnosing atypical symptoms. To our knowledge, no study has demonstrated improved survival from repeat PCI or CABG in any subgroup of post-CABG patients.

2. Approach to cardiac catheterization and bypass graft angiography

The approach to cardiac catheterization in a patient with prior CABG is the same as the approach to cardiac catheterization in patients without CABG for a right heart catheterization, left heart catheterization, and native coronary angiography. Graft arterography includes finding and selectively engaging each graft, usually one LIMA graft and one or more grafts arising from the ascending aorta.

2.1 Pre-catheterization preparation

It is critically important for the operator to know the details of the CABG surgery before starting catheterization, in order to plan access. For example, the best access for a patient with LIMA and RIMA grafts, or with the left radial used for CABG, may be femoral access. It is critically important for the operator to review the operative report because this is the only reliable roadmap to finding grafts. Downstream descriptions of the surgery become progressively unreliable. Specifically, the discharge summary is usually written by an advanced practice provider who may misinterpret the operative report, and subsequent summaries by cardiologists or primary care providers are routinely misleading. For example, a LIMA to the LAD with radial Y-graft to the diagonal and an SVG jumping from the second obtuse marginal to the RCA postero-lateral branch will be recorded in subsequent clinic notes as a 4-vessel CABG. But without details, the operator will not know how many anastomoses from the aorta to look for, or whether a graft will be arising from the right side of the aorta as is typical of grafts to the RCA. When the allowable contrast dose is limited by kidney disease it is particularly important to know details of coronary anatomy to prevent excessive test injections while searching for grafts.

When details of the surgery are unavailable, patients are usually reliable sources of the number of distal anastomoses. Usually, when patients are told the results of their surgery by the surgical team, they are told the number of distal anastomoses, which may exceed the number of proximal anastomoses. The wise operator will make sure all distal anastomoses are accounted for before ending a procedure.

2.2 Vascular access

Radial access decreases vascular complications compared to femoral access in patients without prior CABG. The same is true for patients after CABG, but left radial artery access is preferred since it offers easy access to the origin of the LIMA. In patients with the left radial artery harvested for use as a bypass graft, femoral access is usually used although experienced operators can non-selectively (and occasionally selectively) cannulate the LIMA using right radial access. With left radial access, the left arm can be pulled across the abdomen so the operator does not have to reach across the table. The use of the distal radial access site ("snuffbox approach") can bring the access point even closer to the operator standing on the right side of the table. The RADIAL-CABG randomized trial compared femoral access to left radial access at a single center and demonstrated higher radiation doses, contrast volumes, and longer procedure times with left radial access as compared to femoral access; though radial access was associated with higher patient satisfaction. The crossover rate was higher (17%) in the transradial group compared to the transfemoral group [0%] [10]. A meta-analysis found fewer vascular complications with radial access [11].

2.3 Graft markers

Graft markers are used or not used variably by cardiac surgeons. Common varieties include a small disk usually placed above the aortic anastomosis, a horseshoe or wire ring around the proximal part of the graft, or occasionally just a clip by the aortic anastomosis. Often SVGs or in situ LIMA grafts will have clips where side branch veins were cut; these can lead like breadcrumbs along the course of the graft and give a hint as to the location of its terminus.

2.4 Catheter selection and angiographic views

A typical patient will have a LIMA graft arising from the left subclavian anastomosing distally to the LAD and two or three free grafts, usually SVGs, with anastomoses from the aorta to the target vessel in the LCX system, RCA system, or a diagonal branch of the LAD. Our general approach is described in **Table 1**.

The LIMA is engaged by finding its ostium in the subclavian artery. It may arise on the more proximal vertical section or on the more distal horizontal section of the subclavian. We use the anterior–posterior view although occasionally the right anterior oblique view will better separate the proximal LIMA from the subclavian. From left radial access, the JR4 catheter is advanced over a wire retrograde in the left subclavian to the LIMA ostium. From femoral access, the JR is advanced retrograde through the transverse aorta. Counter-clockwise rotation allows the operator to place the catheter sequentially in the right innominate, then the left carotid, and finally into the left subclavian. The JR4 catheter can be advanced over a wire distally into the

Graft	LIMA to LAD	SVG/ radial to RCA	SVG/ radial to LCX	SVG/radial to Diagonal	RIMA to LCX	In-situ GEA
Catheters	1: JR4 2: IMA 3: VB1	1: Multi A 2: AL1/2 3: BG right	1: JR4 2: AL2 3: Multi 4: BG left	1: JR4 2: AL2 3: Multi 4: BG left	1: JR4 2: IMA 3: VB1	JR4 engages through the hepato-splenic artery
View	AP cranial RAO Left lateral	LAO RAO RAO cranial LAO cranial	LAO RAO AP caudal	LAO cranial LAO RAO	LAO RAO	(Depends on anastomosed artery)

Table 1.
An approach to bypass graft angiography.

subclavian. From either access point, the JR4 can be gently maneuvered proximally in the subclavian with gentle counter-clockwise rotation and test injections. If the origin of the LIMA is acute the JR4 can be exchanged over a wire for an IMA catheter and maneuvered similarly. For a severely angulated LIMA origin, a VB-1 or similar catheter with a pigtail-like curve can be positioned beyond the ostium and pulled back to engage the LIMA ostium (**Table 2**).

Free grafts to the other coronary arteries (i.e. SVGs or radial grafts) are found in the proximal ascending aorta. The grafts are found by selecting a catheter and searching the aorta above the level of the coronary arteries. Right coronary artery grafts will be located on the right side of the aorta whereas left circumflex and diagonal grafts will be located on the left or posterior aspects of the aorta. Generally, grafts are arranged in the following ascending position in the aorta: RCA grafts lowest in the aorta, followed by LAD grafts (if there is SVG to LAD) located a little higher, followed by diagonal branch, then left circumflex first obtuse marginal, second obtuse marginal, and circumflex posterolateral grafts highest in the aorta. We favor multipurpose shapes (or right bypass graft shape) for grafts to the RCA (which usually have a downward takeoff). Grafts to diagonal branches or circumflex branches may be cannulated with the JR or multi-shaped catheter, but if necessary Amplatz-shaped catheters or left bypass graft catheters can be used. For all of these, we use a clockwise rotation of the catheter with frequent test injections to engage grafts.

On occasion, it can be hard to find all of the grafts. When searching for grafts, start with a specific catheter for the suspected graft as described above. A proximally occluded graft may be demonstrated by test injections showing a short stump in a side view or a circle in an end-on view. Occasionally grafts are flush occluded at the aorta and cannot be identified. For RCA grafts it is important to point the catheter downward in the graft using a slight counter-clockwise torque since injection in the proximal graft orthogonal to its direction can mimic a total occlusion. Consider that a graft may arise from an unusual location on the ascending aorta or even from the descending aorta [13], or that a RIMA or gastroepiploic artery may have been used. When all else fails, non-selective aortography can be performed although it does not reliably demonstrate all patent grafts. The last option for finding a graft would be a CT or MRI angiogram.

It may be helpful to identify native vessels that appear to have been grafted. Occasionally the stump of the graft where it is terminally anastomosed to the vessel

Name	Type	Study
GuardWire	Distal balloon	SAFER demonstrated improved rates of periprocedural MI and no-reflow as compared to usual therapy
TriActiv	Distal balloon	PRIDE demonstrated noninferiority to the GuardWire and FilterWire
FilterWire*	Distal filter	FIRE demonstrated noninferiorty to the GuardWire
SpideRx*	Distal filter	SPIDER demonstrated noninferiority to the GuardWire and FilterWire
CardioShield	Distal filter	CAPTIVE failed to demonstrate noninferiority to the GuardWire
Proxis	Proximal balloon	PROXIMAL demonstrated noninferiority to the GuardWire and FilterWire

**Currently available in the USA.*
Source: Lee et al. [12].

Table 2.
Embolic protection devices.

may be seen. In other cases where the graft has flush-occluded, a characteristic upward omega-bend of the native vessel caused by scarring/retraction of the graft after surgery may reveal where the graft was anastomosed to the native vessel. Occasionally a segment of a jump graft between two native branches will remain patent even after the graft from the aorta to the first anastomosis has occluded.

3. Bypass graft PCI

PCI in patients who are post-CABG is common. Data published from the NCDR CathPCI registry in 2011 show that PCI in prior CABG patients represents 17.5% of all PCIs. Native arteries were targeted alone in 62.5% of PCI in prior CABG patients, saphenous vein grafts were the target in 34.9%, and arterial grafts were the target in 2.5% [14]. A similar observational analysis from VA medical centers in 2016 showed overall similar data (73.4% of PCI was in a native artery, 25.0% in an SVG, and 1.5% in an arterial graft). The VA analysis demonstrated that procedure-related complications were more frequent in bypass PCI patients compared to those without, including in-hospital mortality, procedural complications, peri-procedural MI, no-reflow, and dissection. The patients who received PCI to graft lesions were also noted to have higher mortality, MI, and revascularization at 1 and 5 years of follow-up [15].

Indications for PCI in post-CABG patients are similar to those without prior CABG. Graft lesions causing acute coronary syndromes may undergo PCI or may be used as conduits for retrograde PCI of the native vessel to which they anastomose. In stable patients, PCI is generally not indicated for asymptomatic patients. The strength of indication for PCI increases as the severity of symptoms despite guideline medical therapy increases.

3.1 Approach to SVG PCI

There are several issues with intervention on SVGs, and as such, the operator must carefully consider their options before embarking on SVG intervention. SVG intervention carries a high risk of distal embolization, no-reflow, and peri-procedural MI. Degenerated vein grafts are noted in both the ACC/AHA and SCAI classification schemes to be high-risk lesions and to have worse outcomes as compared to low-to-intermediate risk native vessel lesions [16]. Several principles affect decisions regarding SVG intervention.

A first principle of vein graft intervention is that PCI in vein grafts is less reliable than PCI of native coronary arteries. Observational data suggest that PCI to SVGs is associated with worse outcomes than PCI to native coronary arteries [15, 17, 18]. For this reason, when reasonable, restoration of blood flow by performing PCI to the native vessel is preferred to PCI of the SVG. Preferencing PCI to the native artery where possible is given a Class 2a recommendation in the updated 2021 ACC/AHA Coronary Artery Revascularization guidelines [19]. It should be noted that this strategy is complicated by the high rate of CTOs in bypassed native arteries, and referral to a physician with experience in complex coronary disease and CTO may be necessary [20, 21]. A strategy of PCI to the SVG followed by staged PCI to the native artery, especially in the setting of acute MI, may be useful [22]. Intentional iatrogenic occlusion of the SVG after native vessel PCI may be beneficial to reduce competitive flow [23, 24].

A second principle is that intermediate lesions should in general be treated medically. Two trials, VELETI and VELETI II studied the utility of stenting intermediate

SVG lesions. While there was a trend in the VELETI pilot study towards improved outcomes with stenting, the larger VELETI II study showed no benefit [25–27]. Additionally, the use of FFR has been studied in intermediate lesions. While there may be benefit to the use of FFR in arterial grafts, no benefit was seen in SVG lesions and should probably not be used in this setting [28].

A third principle is that PCI to CTOs of SVGs is not of benefit and should not be performed. Chronic total occlusions of SVGs were studied in a retrospective study published in 2010 that found success rate of PCI of SVG CTO was 68%. In the successful PCI group, the ISR rate was 68% and TVR rate was 61% with a median follow up of 18 months [29]. Due to the low success rates and high rate of revascularization, current guidelines give PCI of SVG CTOs a Class 3: No Benefit designation [19].

3.2 Balloons and stents

Bare-metal stenting was clearly an improvement over balloon angioplasty for SVG lesions. The Saphenous Vein in De Novo (SAVED) trial compared bare-metal stents to balloon angioplasty for focal, de-novo SVGs lesions. Stenting increased the procedural success, demonstrating 92% success with BMS versus 69% for angioplasty [30]. This benefit of BMS as compared to balloon angioplasty alone was reinforced with data from the Venestent trial [31].

Several studies have examined the use of bare-metal versus drug-eluting stents in SVG PCI. The RRISC trial initially demonstrated improved outcomes of DES as compared to BMS [32], however the DELAYED RRISC study (a post hoc analysis of the RRISC trial) appeared to support increased mortality of patients treated with DES as compared to BMS [33]. Subsequent randomized controlled trials and meta-analyses have however demonstrated the safety of DES in SVGs [34, 35]. In addition to some smaller trials, two larger RCTs compared DES to BMS: ISAR-CABG and DIVA. While ISAR-CABG did demonstrate lower target lesion revascularization with DES as compared to BMS at 12 months [36], by follow-up at 5 years no difference between DES and BMS was observed [34]. The DIVA trial showed no difference at 12 months between DES and BMS [37]. A meta-analysis of the available RCTs done in 2018 showed no difference between DES and BMS [35]. Of note, in the ISAR-CABG trial, most stents were first-generation, while in the DIVA trial most stents were second-generation indicating that neither first nor second-generation DES stents are an improvement over BMS [35]. Two retrospective studies have found no difference between first- and second-generation DES [38, 39].

Directly stenting SVG lesions (as opposed to performing pre-dilation) might prevent distal embolization. One observational study done in 2003 indicated that direct stenting decreased post-procedural MB-CK elevation, and the one-year composite endpoint of death, Q-wave MI, and target lesion revascularization [40].

Under-sizing stents may improve outcomes in SVG PCI. Hong et al. in 2010 examined a series of patients who underwent SVG PCI with IVUS. They compared patients based on the ratio of stent diameter to vessel diameter and found that patients with relatively under-sized stents had fewer post-procedural CK-MB elevations without worse outcomes at 1 year [41].

3.3 Embolic protection devices

SAFER was a trial in which a distal balloon device called the GuardWire demonstrated a significant decrease in peri-procedural MI and a decrease in no-reflow [42].

The GuardWire is a distal balloon embolic protection device wherein the balloon is inflated distal to the PCI target. The operator then stents the lesion and aspirates the blood containing post-PCI embolic debris out of the vessel before deflating the balloon [42]. The FIRE trial compared a device called the FilterWire, a distal filter-based device, against the GuardWire and showed non-inferiority [43]. Numerous other trials have been investigated (see table below), but all of these trials were in some way compared their device to the GuardWire to show non-inferiority as opposed to a comparison against usual therapy. The TRAP trial would have been a second RCT but was ended due to lack of enrollment and was therefore under-powered; the trend however was of findings consistent with SAFER (decreased peri-procedural MI) [44].

There have been multiple analyses since these trials in the early 2000s looking at EPDs. Iqbal et al. examined the British Columbia Cardiac Registry and showed that patients undergoing SVG PCI had improved post-procedural TIMI flow after EPD use, however had no difference in TVR or mortality at 2 years [45]. Brennan et al. examined the Cath PCI database and showed no difference in rates of death, MI, or TVR with the use of EPDs but did show increased rates of no-reflow, vessel dissection, perforation, and periprocedural MI with the use of EPDs [4]. Paul et al. performed a meta-analysis and review in 2017, which suggested no benefit to EPD use in SVG intervention [46].

The 2011 ACC/AHA guidelines on PCI gave the use of embolic protection devices (EPDs) a Class I recommendation based upon strong randomized control trial evidence from the SAFER trial. However, with the subsequent data described above, current guidelines downgrade the recommendation for use of EPDs from Class I (in 2011) to Class IIa (in 2021) [19, 47]. Despite the data supporting EDP use, estimates of usage rates in SVG lesions based on large registry data range from 14–22% [48, 49]. EPD use may be discouraged by the technical difficulty of using these somewhat bulky devices [49].

In summary, the only randomized trial data available shows the benefit to use of EPD. Multiple other EPDs have shown non-inferiority to the GuardWire. EPDs can be difficult to use which significantly limits their use in clinical practice. And while significant observational data have called into question the findings of the SAFER trial, guideline recommendations are unlikely to change significantly until further RCTs are performed.

3.4 Pharmacology of SVG intervention

In general, antiplatelet drugs are used in the same way post SVG PCI as they would be used post native vessel PCI. The PLATO trial demonstrated the efficacy of ticagrelor over clopidogrel in ACS patients. A post hoc analysis of PLATO showed that ticagrelor was as effective for post-CABG patients as it was for no-CABG patients [50]. In addition, SVG lesions are high-risk lesions and may benefit from more intensive antiplatelet therapy than some native vessel lesions. The DAPT trial showed that in patients who had SVG PCI, there was less stent thrombosis with 30 months of DAPT as compared to 12 months of DAPT [51]. An analysis of the DAPT study developed and validated a prediction rule intended to determine patients who would benefit most from prolonged DAPT. In the generated scoring system, the presence of a vein graft stent was one of the strongest predictors of deriving benefit from prolonged DAPT [24].

The use of GP IIb/IIIa inhibitors does not appear to be of benefit. A meta-analysis of five randomized trials published in 2002 showed that the use of GP IIb/IIIa inhibitors in graft interventions provided no benefit and had an association with worse outcomes [52].

The use of anticoagulants is similar in SVG PCI as in native-vessel PCI. Heparin is the dominant drug used, however, bivalirudin has been shown to be safe and effective [53].

Vasodilator drugs may decrease the rate of no-reflow in SVG PCI. Adenosine, nitroprusside, and the calcium channel blockers verapamil and nicardipine have been investigated. Overall, the quality of the evidence is low however all the studies show some degree of improvement in no-reflow, post-procedural CK-MB elevation, or both in association with the use of vasodilators [54–57]. Nicardipine is often preferred as it causes less hypotension and a longer duration of action [58].

3.5 Other therapeutic options and techniques for SVG

The CORAL trial examined the use of excimer laser coronary atherectomy before stenting. The study failed to enroll enough patients and so they compared laser atherectomy with a stent to the SAFER data (control and EPD groups). The rate of MACE, driven by peri-procedural MI, was lower in the SAFER GuardWire group [59]. One case–control registry indicated that ELCA showed better angiographic outcomes and lower rates of Type IVa MI as compared to distal embolic protection devices [60].

The VeGAS 2 trial compared the AngioJet rheolytic thrombectomy device to urokinase infusion for SVG thrombus. The AngioJet creates a local vacuum using high-velocity water jets, with the intention of sucking thrombus into the catheter for degradation and removal. AngioJet did show some improvements over urokinase infusion, especially in the rates of procedural success, non-Q-wave MI, and vascular complications [61].

3.6 Arterial graft PCI

Arterial grafts are significantly more durable and significantly fewer in number than venous grafts, and they are therefore significantly less likely to be the targets of PCI. PCI in arterial grafts is generally more successful and with lower complication rates than in PCI of vein grafts [14, 15].

The IMA is the most important arterial graft, and there are a few relevant points regarding PCI in these arteries. The risk of complication is not negligible. The most common cause of unsuccessful PCI in an IMA graft is excessive vessel tortuosity. Straightening a tortuous LIMA can cause pseudolesions which may cause ischemia; this effect must be distinguished from vasospasm (as it will not improve with vasodilators) and dissection. Removal of the guidewire should resolve a pseudolesion [58]. Tortuous subclavian arteries may be an issue as well – ipsilateral (usually meaning left) radial access can help in this case. On occasion, coronary ischemia in the distribution of the IMA can be caused by a stenosis of the subclavian artery proximal to the IMA graft, and PCI of the subclavian artery (by an experienced peripheral operator) can relieve the ischemia [62].

Ostial dissections can occur in IMA PCI and therefore the ostium should be evaluated at the end of an IMA PCI procedure. PCI of distal anastomotic IMA lesions has been shown to have better outcomes (less restenosis) with balloon angioplasty as compared to stenting; stents are typically used in lesions of the ostium and the body of IMA grafts [63, 64].

4. Summary

Indications for catheterization and PCI in post-CABG patients are similar to those for patients without CABG. Graft anatomy (taken from the source CABG operative report) should be known before starting a diagnostic procedure. Diagnostic procedures involving grafts are more difficult, require more time, contrast, and catheters, and produce more complications than procedures in patients without prior CABG. A set of unique "tricks" is required to selectively cannulate all grafts known to be present. PCI of grafts, particularly of SVGs, produces frequent complications and is often followed by restenosis. PCI of the native vessel supplying the grafted territory, either antegrade or retrograde, which may be preferred over graft arteriography. As the incidence of CABG is decreasing over recent decades, the number of post-CABG patients undergoing catheterization is decreasing. However, the ability to perform angiography of post-CABG patients will continue as a required skill of invasive interventional cardiologists.

Author details

Reed M. Otten* and James Blankenship
Division of Cardiology, University of New Mexico Health Science Center, Albuquerque, NM, Mexico

*Address all correspondence to: rotten@salud.unm.edu

References

[1] Gaudino M et al. Association of radial artery graft vs saphenous vein graft with long-term cardiovascular outcomes among patients undergoing coronary artery bypass grafting: A systematic review and meta-analysis. JAMA. 2020;**324**(2):179-187

[2] Beerkens FJ et al. Contemporary coronary artery bypass graft surgery and subsequent percutaneous revascularization. Nature Reviews. Cardiology. 2021:1-14

[3] Cho KR, Kim J-S, Choi J-S, Kim K-B. Serial angiographic follow-up of grafts one year and five years after coronary bypass graft surgery. European Journal of Cardio-Thoracic Surgery. 2006;**29**:511-516

[4] Brennan JM, Al-Hejily W, Dai D, et al. Three-year outcomes associated with embolic protection in saphenous vein graft intervention: Results in 49 325 senior patients in the Medicare-linked National Cardiovascular Data Registry CathPCI Registry. Circulation: Cardiovascular Interventions. 2015;**8**(3):e001403

[5] Dimitrova KR, Hoffman DM, Geller CM, Dincheva G, Ko W, Tranbaugh RF. Arterial grafts protect the native coronary vessels from atherosclerotic disease progression. The Annals of Thoracic Surgery. 2012;**94**(2):475-481

[6] Xenogiannis I et al. Saphenous venous graft failure: From pathophysiology to prevention and treatment strategies. Circulation. 2021;**144**:728-745

[7] Patel MR, Bailey SR, Bonow RO, Chambers CE, Chan PS, Dehmer GJ, et al. ACCF/SCAI/AATS/AHA/ASE/ASNC/HFSA/HRS/SCCM/SCCT/SCMR/STS 2012 appropriate use criteria for diagnostic catheterization: A report of the American College of Cardiology Foundation Appropriate Use Criteria Task Force, Society for Cardiovascular Angiography and Interventions, American Association for Thoracic Surgery, American Heart Association, American Society of Echocardiography, American Society of Nuclear Cardiology, Heart Failure Society of America, Heart Rhythm Society, Society of Critical Care Medicine, Society of Cardiovascular Computed Tomography, Society for Cardiovascular Magnetic Resonance, and Society of Thoracic Surgeons. Journal of the American College of Cardiology. 2012;**59**(22):1995-2027. DOI: 10.1016/j.jacc.2012.03.003

[8] Thielmann M, Sharma V, Al-Attar N, Bulluck H, Bisleri G, Bunge JJH, et al. ESC Joint Working Groups on Cardiovascular Surgery and the Cellular Biology of the Heart position paper: Perioperative myocardial injury and infarction in patients undergoing coronary artery bypass graft surgery. European Heart Journal. 2017;**38**:2392-2407

[9] Thygesen K et al. Fourth Universal Definition of Myocardial Infarction (2018). Journal of the American College of Cardiology. 2018;**72**(18):2231-2264

[10] Tesfaldet MT et al. A Randomized Comparison of the Transradial and Transfemoral Approaches for Coronary Artery Bypass Graft Angiography and Intervention: The RADIAL-CABG Trial (RADIAL Versus Femoral Access for Coronary Artery Bypass Graft Angiography and Intervention). JACC: Cardiovascular Intervention. **6**(11):1138-1144

[11] Rigattieri S et al. Meta-analysis of radial versus femoral artery approach

for coronary procedures in patients with previous coronary artery bypass grafting. The American Journal of Cardiology. 2016;**117**:1248e1255

[12] Lee MS et al. Saphenous vein graft intervention. Journal of American College of Cardiology. 2011;**4**:831-843

[13] Baker NC et al. Left radial artery access to a descending aortic saphenous vein graft to circumflex coronary artery for angioplasty. The Journal of Invasive Cardiology. 2012;**24**(7):352-353

[14] Brilakis ES et al. Percutaneous coronary intervention in native arteries versus bypass grafts in prior coronary artery bypass grafting patients. Journal of American Cardiology. 2011;**4**:844-850

[15] Brilakis ES et al. Percutaneous coronary intervention in native coronary arteries versus bypass grafts in patients with prior coronary artery bypass graft surgery: Insights from the veterans affairs clinical assessment, reporting, and tracking program. Journal of American Cardiology. 2016;**9**:884-893

[16] Krone et al. A simplified lesion classification for predicting success and complications of coronary angiography. The American Journal of Cardiology. 2000;**85**:1179-1184

[17] Hoffman R et al. Implantation of sirolimus-eluting stents in saphenous vein grafts is associated with high clinical follow-up event rates compared with treatment of native vessels. Coronary Artery Disease. 2007;**18**:559-564

[18] Redfors B et al. Percutaneous coronary intervention of saphenous vein graft. Circulation: Cardiovascular Interventions. 2017;**10**:e004953

[19] Lawton JS et al. 2021 ACC/AHA/SCAI Guideline for coronary artery revascularization: A report of the american college of cardiology/American heart association joint committee on clinical practice guidelines. Journal of the American College of Cardiology. 2022;**79**(2):e21-e129

[20] Riley R et al. SCAI position statement on optimal percutaneous coronary interventional therapy for complex coronary artery disease. Catheterization and Cardiovascular Interventions. 2020;**96**:346-362

[21] Brilakis ES, Banerjee S, Burke MN. New treatment strategy for saphenous vein graft lesions?: Letting it go. Journal of the American College of Cardiology. 2018;**71**(18):1983-1985

[22] Xenogiannis I, Tajti P, Burke MN, Brilakis ES. Staged revascularization in patients with acute coronary syndromes due to saphenous vein graft failure and chronic total occlusion of the native vessel: A novel concept. Catheterization and Cardiovascular Interventions. 2019;**93**(3):440-444

[23] Wilson SJ et al. Saphenous vein graft sacrifice following native vessel PCI is safe and associated with favourable longer-term outcomes. Cardiovascular Revascularization Medicine. 2019;**20**:1048-1052

[24] Yeh RW, Secemsky EA, Kereiakes DJ, et al. Development and validation of a prediction rule for benefit and harm of dual antiplatelet therapy beyond 1 year after percutaneous coronary intervention. Journal of the American Medical Association. 2016;**315**(16):1735-1749

[25] Rodés-Cabau J, Bertrand OF, Larose E, Déry JP, Rinfret S, Bagur R, et al. Comparison of plaque sealing with paclitaxel-eluting stents versus medical therapy for the treatment of

moderate non-significant saphenous vein graft lesions: The moderate vein graft lesion stenting with the taxus stent and intravascular ultrasound (VELETI) pilot trial. Circulation. 2009;**120**:1978-1986. DOI: 10.1161/CIRCULATIONAHA.109.874057

[26] Rodés-Cabau J, Bertrand OF, Larose E, Déry JP, Rinfret S, Urena M, et al. Five-year follow-up of the plaque sealing with paclitaxel-eluting stents vs medical therapy for the treatment of intermediate nonobstructive saphenous vein graft lesions (VELETI) trial. The Canadian Journal of Cardiology. 2014;**30**:138-145. DOI: 10.1016/j.cjca.2013.11.002

[27] Rodes-Cabau J, Jolly SS, Cairns J, Mansour S, L'Allier PL, Teefy PJ, et al. Sealing intermediate nonobstruc- tive coronary saphenous vein graft lesions with drug-eluting stents as a new approach to reducing cardiac events: A randomized controlled trial. Circulation. Cardiovascular Interventions. 2016;**9**:e004336

[28] Di Serafino L, De Bruyne B, Mangiacapra F, et al. Long-term clinical outcome after fractional flow reserve-versus angio-guided percutaneous coronary intervention in patients with intermediate stenosis of coronary artery bypass grafts. American Heart Journal. 2013;**166**:110-118

[29] Al-Lamee R et al. Clinical and angiographic outcomes after percutaneous recanalization of chronic total saphenous vein graft occlusion using modern techniques. Journal of Cardiology. 2010;**106**:1721-1727

[30] Savage MP, Douglas JS, Fischman DL, Pepine CJ, King SB, Werner JA, et al. Stent placement compared with balloon angioplasty for obstructed coronary bypass grafts. The New England Journal of Medicine. 1997;**337**:740-747

[31] Hanekamp CEE, Koolen JJ, den Heijer P, Schalij MJ, Piek JJ, Bar FWHM, et al. Randomized study to compare balloon angioplasty and elective stent implantation in venous bypass grafts: The Venestent study. Catheterization and Cardiovascular Interventions. 2003;**60**:452-457

[32] Vermeersch P, Agostoni P, Verheye S, et al. Randomized double-blind comparison of sirolimus-eluting stent versus bare metal stent implantation in diseased saphenous vein grafts: Six-month angiographic, intravascular ultrasound, and clinical follow-up of the RRISC trial. Journal of the American College of Cardiology. 2006;**48**:2423-2431

[33] Vermeersch P, Agostini P, Verheye S, Van den Heuvel P, Convens C, Van den Branden F, et al. Increased late mortality after sirolimus-eluting stents versus bare-metal stents in diseased sahenous vein grafts: Results from the randomized DELAYED RRISC Trial. Journal of the American College of Cardiology. 2007

[34] Colleran R et al. Efficacy over time with drug-eluting stents in saphenous vein graft lesions. Journal of the American College of Cardiology. 2018;**71**:1973-1982

[35] Patel et al. Drug-eluting stents versus bare-metal stents in saphenous vein graft intervention: An updated meta-analysis of randomized controlled trials. Circulation. Cardiovascular Interventions. 2018;**11**:e007045

[36] Mehilli J et al. Drug-eluting versus bare-metal stents in saphenous vein graft lesions (ISAR-CABG): A randomised controlled superiority trial. The Lancet. 2011;**378**:1071-1178

[37] Brilakis ES et al. Drug-eluting stents versus bare-metal stents in saphenous

vein grafts: A double-blind, randomised trial. Lancet. 2018;**391**:1997-2007

[38] Polaka NR et al. Long-term outcomes with first- vs. second-generation drug-eluting stents in saphenous vein graft lesions. Catheterization and Cardiovascular Interventions. 2016;**87**:34-40

[39] Costopoulos C et al. Comparison of first- and second-generation drug-eluting stents in saphenous vein grafts used as aorto-coronary conduits. The American Journal of Cardiology. 2013;**112**:318e322

[40] Leborgne L, Cheneau E, Pichard A, Ajani A, Pakala R, Yazdi H, et al. Effect of direct stenting on clinical outcome in patients treated with percutaneous coronary intervention on saphenous vein graft. American Heart Journal. 2003;**146**:501-506

[41] Hong YJ, Pichard AD, Mintz GS, et al. Outcome of undersized drug- eluting stents for percutaneous coronary intervention of saphenous vein graft lesions. The American Journal of Cardiology. 2010;**105**(2):179-185

[42] Baim DS, Wahr D, George B, Leon MB, Greenberg J, Cutlip DE, et al. Randomized trial of a distal embolic protection device during percutaneous intervention of saphenous vein aorto-coronary bypass grafts. Circulation. 2002;**105**:1285-1290

[43] Stone GW, Rogers C, Hermiller J, Feldman R, Hall P, Haber R, et al. Randomized comparison of distal protection with a filter-based catheter and a balloon occlusion and aspiration system during percutaneous intervention of diseased saphenous vein aorto-coronary bypass grafts. Circulation. 2003;**108**:548-553

[44] Dixon SR et al. A Randomized, Controlled Trial of Saphenous Vein Graft Intervention with a Filter-Based Distal Embolic Protection Device: TRAP Trial. Journal of Interventional Cardiology. 2005;**18**:233-241

[45] Iqbal MB et al. Embolic protection device use and its association with procedural safety and long-term outcomes following saphenous vein graft intervention: An analysis from the British Columbia cardiac registry. Catheterization and Cardiovascular Interventions. 2016;**88**:73-83

[46] Paul TK, Bhatheja S, Panchal HB, et al. Outcomes of saphenous vein graft intervention with and without embolic protection device: A comprehensive review and meta-analysis. Circulation: Cardiovascular Interventions. 2017;**10**(12):e005538

[47] Levine GN et al. 2011 ACCF/AHA/SCAI Guideline for Percutaneous Coronary Intervention: A Report of the American College of Cardiology Foundation/American Heart Association Task Force on Practice Guidelines and the Society for Cardiovascular Angiography and Interventions. Journal of the American College of Cardiology. Dec 2011;**58**(24):e44-e122

[48] Mehta SK, Frutkin AD, Milford-Beland S, et al. Utilization of distal embolic protection in saphenous vein graft interventions (an analysis of 19,546 patients in the American College of Cardiology-National Cardiovascular Data Registry). The American Journal of Cardiology. 2007;**100**(7):1114-1118

[49] Shoaib A et al. Outcomes following percutaneous coronary intervention in saphenous vein grafts with and without embolic protection devices. JACC: Cardiovascular Interventions. 2019;**12**:2286-2295

[50] Brilakis ES, Held C, Meier B, Cools F, Claeys MJ, Cornel JH, et al. Effect of

ticagrelor on the outcomes of patients with prior coronary artery bypass graft surgery: Insights from the PLATelet inhibition and patient outcomes (PLATO) trial. American Heart Journal. 2013;**166**(3):474-480

[51] Mauri L, Kereiakes DJ, Yeh RW, et al. Twelve or 30 months of dual antiplatelet therapy after drug-eluting stents. The New England Journal of Medicine. 2014;**371**:2155-2166

[52] Roffi M, Mukherjee D, Chew DP, Bhatt DL, Cho L, Robbins MA, et al. Lack of benefit from intravenous platelet glycoprotein IIb/IIIa receptor inhibition as adjunctive treatment for percutaneous interventions of aortocoronary bypass grafts: A pooled analysis of five randomized clinical trials. Circulation. 2002;**106**:3063-3067. DOI: 10.1161/01.cir.0000041250.89627.a9

[53] Kao J, Lincoff AM, Topol EJ, Madrid A, Price J, Sawhney M, et al. Direct thrombin inhibition appears to be a safe and effective anticoagulant for percutaneous bypass graft interventions. Catheterization and Cardiovascular Interventions. 2006;**68**:352-356

[54] Fischell TA, Subraya RG, Ashraf K, Perry B, Haller S. "Pharmacologic" distal protection using prophylactic, intragraft nicardipine to prevent no-reflow and non-Q-wave myocardial infarction during elective saphenous vein graft intervention. The Journal of Invasive Cardiology. 2007;**19**:58-62

[55] Michaels AD, Appleby M, Otten MH, et al. Pretreatment with intra- graft verapamil prior to percutaneous coronary intervention of saphenous vein graft lesions: Results of the randomized, controlled vasodilator prevention on no-reflow (VAPOR) trial. The Journal of Invasive Cardiology. 2002;**14**(6):299-302

[56] Zoghbi GJ, Goyal M, Hage F, et al. Pretreatment with nitroprusside for microcirculatory protection in saphenous vein graft interventions. The Journal of Invasive Cardiology. 2009;**21**(2):34-39

[57] Sdringola S, Assali A, Ghani M, et al. Adenosine use during aortocoronary vein graft interventions reverses but does not prevent the slow-no reflow phenomenon. Catheterization and Cardiovascular Interventions. 2000;**51**(4):394-399

[58] Xenogiannis I, Tajti P, Hall AB, Alaswad K, Rinfret S, Nicholson W, et al. Update on cardiac catheterization in patients with prior coronary artery bypass graft surgery. JACC. Cardiovascular Interventions. 2019;**12**:1635-1649. DOI: 10.1016/j.jcin.2019.04.051

[59] Giugliano GR et al. A prospective multicenter registry of laser therapy for degenerated saphenous vein graft stenosis: The COronary graft Results following Atherectomy with Laser (CORAL) trial. Cardiovascular Revascularization Medicine. 2012;**13**:84-89

[60] Niccoli G et al. Case-control registry of excimer laser coronary angioplasty versus distal protection devices in patients with acute coronary syndromes due to saphenous vein graft disease. The American Journal of Cardiology. 2013;**112**:1586e1591

[61] Kuntz RE et al. A Trial Comparing Rheolytic Thrombectomy With Intracoronary Urokinase for Coronary and Vein Graft Thrombus (The Vein Graft AngioJet Study [VeGAS 2]). The American Journal of Cardiology. 2002;**89**:326-330

[62] Dimas B et al. ST-segment elevation acute myocardial infarction due to severe hypotension and proximal left subclavian artery stenosis in a prior

coronary artery bypass graft patient. Cardiovascular Revascularization Medicine. 2009;**10**:191-194

[63] Kockeritz U et al. Results of angioplasty (with or without stent) at the site of the narrowed coronary anastomosis of the left internal mammary artery graft or via the internal mammary artery. The American Journal of Cardiology. 2004;**93**:1531-1533

[64] Gruberg L et al. Percutaneous revascularization of the internal mammary artery graft: Short- and long-term outcomes. Journal of the American College of Cardiology. 2000;**35**:944-948

Chapter 3

Perioperative Glycemic Control for Patients Undergoing Coronary Artery Bypass Grafting

Cheng Luo, Chuan Wang, Xiaoyong Xie and BaoShi Zheng

Abstract

Coronary artery bypass grafting (CABG), as a gold standard treatment for coronary artery disease, has been widely adopted all around the world. Meanwhile, it's also well known that diabetes is an independent risk factor for postoperative mortality. However, hyperglycemia often occurs perioperatively, regardless of whether the patient has diabetes or not. Perioperative stress hyperglycemia is harmful to patients undergoing cardiac surgery and has a clear correlation with increased inflammatory response, and clinical adverse events, especially for patients with diabetes. Thus, proper perioperative blood glycemic control can reduce the short-term and long-term mortality and the incidence of complications in patients undergoing CABG.

Keywords: coronary artery disease, diabetes mellitus, mortality, complications, glycemic control

1. Introduction

With the development of society and environment, the number of patients with coronary artery disease (CAD) is increasing, and a large number of patients have diffuse CAD, especially in patients with diabetes. Conservative treatment or interventional therapy is difficult to achieve satisfying results. Coronary artery bypass grafting (CABG) plays an irreplaceable role in the treatment of cardiovascular disease, but with larger trauma requiring thoracotomy. It is easy to develop stress hyperglycemia in both diabetic patients and non-diabetic patients. Previous studies have proved that hyperglycemia is an independent risk factor for increased postoperative mortality and complications. In addition to primary lesions, the risk of cardiovascular complications caused by diabetes may increase by 2–4 times. About 5.2% of CABG patients may have diabetes without preoperative diagnosis. Perioperative glycemic control also affects the prognosis of CABG, as a result, it is important for most patients to control blood glucose regardless of whether they are diagnosed with diabetes.

2. Mechanism of hyperglycemia after CABG

Cardiac surgery is prone to stress response, which is mainly caused by the massive release of neuroendocrine hormones, high catabolism, heat production and hyperglycemia. Diabetic patients suffer from insulin resistance (IR) due to the loss of sensitivity to insulin at physiological level. The intensive stress reaction increases IR after operation, which is characterized by pathological hyperglycemia, impaired glucose tolerance, increased lipolysis and hyperinsulinemia, which may cause a series of metabolic disorders and increased burden on the heart and lungs [1]. In addition to hyperglycemia, IR also has an impact on fat and amino acid metabolism by accelerating its catabolism and presents with clinical hyperlipidemia and negative nitrogen balance. Postoperative IR is a special metabolic state similar to type 2 diabetes after operation. The body's biological response to insulin is weaker than normal, and it can also occur in patients with elective surgery without diabetes. Stress hyperglycemia (SH) is an independent risk factor affecting the prognosis and is directly related to the poor prognosis of elderly patients who underwent cardiac surgery [2]. During the CABG operation, whether patients are diabetic or undergoing cardiopulmonary bypass (CPB), especially in the absence of exogenous insulin, significant increases in blood glucose may occur, leading to various causes of hyperglycemia.

2.1 Surgical trauma

CABG with thoracotomy is a great stimulus, which may cause the hormone levels to lose balance, resulting in reactive hyperglycemia. The operation process will directly promote the production of some stress hormones (such as catecholamine, glucocorticoid, glucagon and growth hormone), in which the secretion of glucocorticoid is more than 10 times higher than usual. These are antagonistic hormones of insulin, which can promote glycogenolysis, liver gluconeogenesis, fat and protein catabolism, while inhibiting insulin release, reducing tissue sensitivity to insulin and increasing peripheral tissues' IR, and thus, leads to a decreased glucose utilization, increased liver glycogen output and increased blood glucose reactivity [3]. The surgery process can also promote the production of a large number of cytokines and inflammatory mediators (such as tumour necrosis factor, interleukin-1 and interleukin-6), which will increase the secretion of the above stress hormones, resulting in decreased insulin secretion, increased IR and impaired glucose utilization, resulting in reactive hyperglycemia. Due to the decreased responsiveness and sensitivity of peripheral tissues to insulin, patients with surgical stress reactions cannot generate normal biological effects under a normal dose of insulin, with the IR and hyperglycemia coexisting with hyperinsulinemia [4]. It is generally believed that the molecular biological mechanism of IR is related to abnormal pre insulin receptor function, disorders of post insulin receptor signal transduction, glucose transport, intracellular metabolism and inflammation cytokines (such as tumour necrosis factor).

2.2 SH produced by CPB

Coronary artery disease (CAD) complicated with valve disease and other heart diseases usually requires revascularization under CPB, and factors such as hypothermia, hypotension, hemodilution, non-pulsatile perfusion and anaesthesia may cause strong stimulation during the surgery. The resulting strong reaction can increase the concentration of glucose, free fatty acids, glycerol and lactic acid in blood, inhibit the phosphorylation of insulin in peripheral tissue cells, insulin receptor substrate-1 and cell division activated protein kinase and produce IR and abnormal glucose tolerance [5]. At the same time, the increase of adrenocortical hormone caused by stress can also indirectly aggravate hyperglycemia and IR. The mechanisms are as follows: (1) pre receptor: increased secretion of catecholamine, growth hormone, cortisol and glucagon to resist the hypoglycemic effect of insulin; (2) receptor: the down-regulation of the number of receptors and the decrease of the binding rate between insulin and receptors; (3) Post receptor: the activity of insulin substrate decreases and the number of glucose transporters decreases. In addition, a series of stimulation of CPB can promote the generation of endogenous blood glucose, reduce the uptake of blood glucose by tissues, and strengthen the reabsorption of glucose filtered in original urine by kidneys, so as to increase blood glucose.

CPB aggravates postoperative IR in patients with CABG and increases glycemia in both diabetic and nondiabetic patients [6]. It makes glycemic control more difficult in the early postoperative period, which is significantly associated with early mortality and morbidity. For patients with diabetes mellitus and poor coronary artery condition, it is off-pump CABG operation (which performs CABG without CPB) might be an alternative option. Meanwhile, surgeons should always pay attention to the risk and risk factors of postoperative hyperglycemia and insulin resistance and reduce insulin resistance and postoperative blood glucose level to promote postoperative recovery.

2.3 Psychosocial factors

In addition to physical stress, patients also have psychosocial stress perioperatively, such as fear or even anxiety. As a result, a series of physiological changes (such as rapid heartbeat, increased sweating, etc.) will occur, which may be caused by the increased excitability of sympathetic nerve and the imbalance of autonomic nervous system. Sympathetic nerve excitation will lead to the increased secretion of glucocorticoids such as adrenal hormone, which will increase blood glucose. Therefore, the psychological state is also an important factor affecting the perioperative blood glucose stability, and it plays an important role in the occurrence and development of SH.

2.4 Other factors

Topical drugs during surgery are also one of the factors leading to SH, such as catecholamines, cyclosporine, steroids, diuretics, protein inhibitors, growth hormone, etc. These drugs can also affect glucose metabolism and cause reactive hyperglycemia.

3. The danger of hyperglycemia

3.1 Damage to heart

Hyperglycemia damages almost all organs, especially the heart. The study found that the incidence of postoperative complications of non-diabetic patients with unsatisfactory glycemic control was significantly higher than that of patients with ideal glycemic control, and the prognosis was even worse. SH will affect the immunity of patients undergoing cardiovascular surgery and reduce the anti-infection ability.

SH can not only inhibit the phagocytosis and chemotaxis of autoimmune cells and neutrophils but also destroy the structure of cells and increase the permeability of cell wall, thus affecting the function of cells [7]. SH makes the blood become viscous, with red blood cells and platelets gathered, causing blood hypercoagulability and gradually forming thrombosis. Free radicals aggravate oxidation, produce a large number of lipid peroxides in the blood and adhere to the vessel wall, making the blood vessel cavity thinner, the pipe wall rough, the elasticity weaker and the blood vessel brittle, thus increasing the incidence of cardiovascular events. It is found that the level of blood glucose is positively correlated with the size of myocardial infarction area [8]. The higher the blood glucose level is, the higher the infarct size is. The damage of SH to the heart is mainly manifested in the following aspects.

3.1.1 Increase inflammatory response

In 2002, Esposito et al. reported that in the experiment of healthy patients and diabetics or patients with impaired glucose tolerance, the increase of stress blood glucose could lead to a sharp increase in inflammatory markers and increase the release of inflammatory factors, thereby aggravating the inflammatory response. In 2003, marfella et al. found that SH was positively correlated with enhanced inflammatory immune response and could worsen cardiac function. All the above show that SH can exacerbate inflammatory response and reduce cardiac function.

3.1.2 Aggravate the edema of ischemic cardiomyocytes

During CPB, the myocardial ischemia and hypoxia are more obvious, which accelerates the anaerobic glycolysis of glucose, resulting in the increase of the end products of lactic acid, and the permeability of the vascular wall, and thus, forming the edema with the retention of sodium and water [9]. Meanwhile, hyperglycemia also slows down the recovery of calcium ions, resulting in a large amount of calcium ions accumulation in cells, interfering with the process of mitochondrial oxidative phosphorylation, causing disorders of cellular protein and lipid metabolism, and inhibition of sodium and potassium pump. This obstacles of ATP production, and further aggravates the edema of ischemic cardiomyocytes.

3.1.3 Cause decreased cardiac function

SH can reduce cardiac function. Previous studies pointed out that hyperglycemia is significantly related to heart failure and is the main factor affecting the prognosis [10]. When the body is in a state of stress, SH can aggravate myocardial cell injury, increase infarct area, and weaken myocardial contractility with an expansion of necrotic area and ventricle, resulting in ventricular remodelling and increased myocardial oxygen consumption, and further aggravating myocardial ischemia and the risk of heart failure. A remarkable increase in blood glucose caused by excessive stress can lead to the change of hemodynamics, the increase of blood viscosity, aggravating the ischemia and the cardiac insufficiency.

3.2 Effect on prognosis of CABG

Diabetes mellitus (DM) has resulted in an increase in mortality after CABG. The mortality rate of patients without history of diabetes but with perioperative hyperglycemia is also increased. The results of several studies on different glycemic control schemes show that the occurrence of intraoperative and postoperative hyperglycemia is positively correlated with the postoperative mortality [11], whether, patients undergo CPB or not during CABG. Blood glucose > 270 mg/dl during CPB is defined as hyperglycemia. The general treatment is a single injection of insulin. However, there is no standardized scheme. For diabetic and non-diabetic patients, intraoperative hyperglycemia is an independent predictor of morbidity and mortality. Relevant studies have shown that if the blood glucose for four consecutive measurements are all > 200 mg/dl, then the glycemic control effect is defined as poor. Compared with patients without hyperglycemia during operation, it can increase the in-hospital mortality and prolong the stay in ICU. Another study confirmed that the average and maximum blood glucose during CABG is one of the independent predictors of short-term postoperative mortality [12]. The average blood glucose during CABG is an important predictor of mortality, pulmonary and renal complications, and it increases the risk of retrosternal wound infection; Meanwhile, DM before CABG is an important risk factor for mortality.

3.3 Complications related to hyperglycemia

Elevated blood glucose will cause changes in body fluid osmotic pressure and affect cell function. The most important effect of hyperglycemia is perioperative infection. Many studies have shown that patients who underwent CABG complicated with hyperglycemia have a significantly increased risk of serious infection, including not only surgical process-related infections (mediastinal infection and wound infection) (**Figure 1**), but also urinary tract infections [13]. Diabetic patients are more likely to develop these complications. The risk of infection after CABG is 4 times higher in patients with DM. Although the specific reasons for the increased risk of infection are not yet clear, this may be related to chronic diseases. For example,

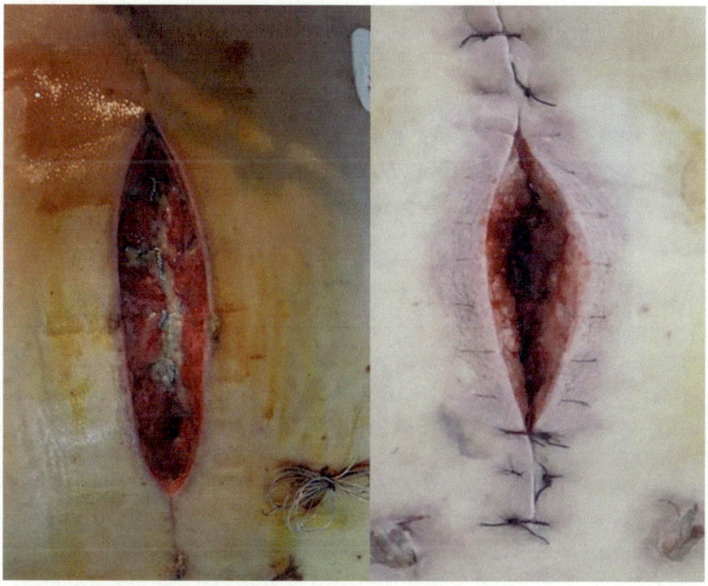

Figure 1.
Poor wound healing after CABG in diabetic patients.

long-term hyperglycemia leads to disorders of the immune system and local hypoxia caused by small vessel diseases. Other studies have also shown that the complications of infection in patients with postoperative hyperglycemia may be based on acute and reversible immune dysfunction, including the weakening of polynuclear bacteriophage and bactericidal effect [14]. Continuous insulin infusion for 24 hours postoperatively can restore the leukocyte function to the baseline level. It has been confirmed that postoperative hyperglycemia will reduce the chemotaxis, conditioning and overall antioxidant effect of lobulated nuclear leukocytes. Although the optimal dose and timing of insulin are unclear, insulin injection can reverse the changes in the immune system.

4. Glycemic control

4.1 Management of perioperative hyperglycemia

Compared with standard insulin therapy, continuous perioperative insulin infusion in cardiac surgery can significantly reduce the mortality by 57%, especially in patients with confirmed hyperglycemia. Lazar et al. found that the GIK of glucose + insulin + potassium before and 12 hours after operation can improve myocardial metabolism [15]. There was no significant difference in the 30-day mortality rate between the study group (glycemic control target at 6.9–11.1 mmol/l) and the control group (glycemic control <13.9 mmol/L), but the 2-year survival rate increased significantly. Lecomte et al. found that intensive glycemic control can reduce the 30-day mortality rate in patients without DM [16]. Most scholars believe that the target blood glucose level of cardiac surgery should be more restrictive.

4.2 Preoperative glycemic control

Preoperative blood glucose level includes fasting blood glucose level at admission, HbA1c level and average fasting blood glucose level 3 days before operation, which has different effects on mortality and cardiovascular-related adverse events. Schmeltz et al. found that the 30-day mortality rate of patients with DM after CABG was 2 times higher than that of non-diabetic patients, but there was no significant correlation between postoperative blood glucose and mortality [17]. Faritus et al. showed that the higher the HbA1c level before CABG, the higher the risk of incidence of postoperative infections [18].

4.3 Intraoperative glycemic control

Schwarzer et al. noticed that the increase of blood glucose during CPB cardiac surgery is an independent predictor of mortality during hospitalization [19]. With the increase of every 1 mmol/L, the mortality rate of diabetic patients will increase by 20%, while the mortality of non-diabetic patients will increase by 12%. The study also showed that when blood glucose was > 5.6 mmol/l, the postoperative adverse events increased by 34% for every 1 mmol/L increase in blood glucose. Ouattara et al. found that poor glycemic control during operation can increase 6.2 times of adverse events during hospitalization. The ideal method of intraoperative glycemic control remains unclear. Related studies showed that intensive insulin therapy did not reduce the time of hospitalization or ICU stay in patients with CAD combined with diabetes, and the effect of intraoperative intensive insulin therapy had no obvious advantage compared with that of postoperative intensive insulin (PII) therapy.

4.4 Postoperative glycemic control

Postoperative stress hyperglycemia can significantly increase the mortality and adverse cardiovascular events. Related studies showed that severe hyperglycemia within 24 hours after CABG was significantly correlated with in-hospital mortality. In 2012, Desai et al. completed the prospective randomized controlled trials of insulin treatment for severe patients [20]. The results showed that PII treatment can reduce the mortality rate within one year, and can significantly reduce the mortality of patients with more than 5 days in ICU. In addition, it is also conducive to improving the quality of life. Meanwhile, PII reduced the incidence of hematogenous infection by 46%, the incidence of dialysis and hemofiltration by 41%, the average transfusion volume by 50%, and the incidence of severe multiple neuropathies by 44%. The results also found that in ICU, the treatment scheme of glycemic control in the surgical group and the non-surgical group treated with drugs brought significantly different results. Similar studies have shown that PII therapy can reduce the mortality of ICU patients, but no significant results were found for simple diabetic patients with the intensive insulin therapy. For diabetic patients, intensive insulin therapy can reduce the incidence of complications, including acute kidney injury and multiple neurological diseases. However, it is still lacking supportive data for the ideal control target of blood glucose as well as the therapy.

5. Perioperative intensive insulin therapy

5.1 Intensive insulin therapy after CABG

Based on the results of the above research and the understanding of the risk factors related to hyperglycemia and hypoglycemia, many perioperative insulin treatment schemes for CABG patients have been proposed. Although these data come from different patient groups, there is a consensus that it is beneficial to closely monitor blood glucose levels and optimize blood glucose data. Due to the different treatment schemes obtained from various literature and research projects, it is difficult to determine the ideal treatment scheme for glycemic control in patients undergoing CABG. Some studies only recommend the treatment guidelines for glycemic control in ICU patients after cardiothoracic surgery, while others provide specific schemes for hyperglycemia treatment. In these studies, a targeted program has successfully reduced the incidence of hypoglycemia [20]. Although some studies have shown that intensive glycemic control is reasonable and the occurrence of hypoglycemic events can be minimized through close glycemic control, no study can provide a specific treatment scheme for clinical use. Most patients use glucose injection and insulin injection to maintain it in a predetermined range by adjusting the injection ratio. Most studies reported that the adjustment of the predetermined blood glucose range reduced the incidence of hypoglycemia, and the commonly recommended blood glucose range was 100–150 mg/dl. In order to achieve the goal, blood glucose must be closely monitored in the operating room and ICU, and it is often required to measure blood glucose at the bedside every hour. Insulin injection therapy is very labour-consuming to monitor and adjust insulin dose at the same time, especially when strictly controlling blood glucose. Therefore, we should determine the individualized blood glucose level and formulate corresponding treatment principles to avoid hypoglycemia.

5.2 Intensive insulin therapy and inflammatory response

CABG under CPB is a clinically mature surgical method. With the continuous improvement of cardiovascular surgical technology and CPB, although the mortality of cardiac surgery has been greatly reduced, various stimulating factors often cause strong stress responses during CPB. It can not only produce stress hyperglycemia but also activate the complement system, resulting in the release of a large number of inflammatory factors, causing systemic inflammatory response syndrome (SIRS), accompanied by typical myocardial haemorrhage and reperfusion injury. SIRS is a self-amplifying and self-destructive inflammatory reaction. If its development is unbalanced, it can induce acute respiratory distress syndrome and multiple organ failure, which are important causes of mortality. A large number of clinical data show that intensive insulin therapy can not only effectively control blood glucose, but also significantly reduce the release of postoperative inflammatory factors, so as to reduce the incidence and mortality of clinical related complications, improve the prognosis of patients and accelerate the rehabilitation.

6. Objectives of glycemic control

Previous studies showed that the risk of infection in patients with postoperative blood glucose>12.2 mmoi/l were 5 times higher than those with normal blood glucose. Once the postoperative blood glucose exceeds the normal level, it should be given hypoglycemic treatment, and it is more appropriate to control the blood glucose in the range of 4.0–6.1 mmoi/l, which can effectively reduce a series of complications caused by hyperglycemia [21]. The increase of postoperative complications can affect or prolong the rehabilitation and hospital stay. Poor postoperative glycemic control will not only affect the healing but also increase the psychological and economic burden of patients. Insulin can be reasonably used to effectively control blood glucose before tracheal intubation is removed after operation. Patients who can eat after extubation can choose appropriate hypoglycemic drugs according to their condition to promote their rehabilitation. According to the results of Leuven Trail in 2001, intensive insulin control of blood glucose in ICU patients (< 6.1 mmol/l) can reduce the risk of death by 42% and the risk of related complications [22]. NICE-SUGAR study in 2009 is the largest multicenter study in ICU patients with intensive glycemic control [23]. The glycemic control goal of this study is < 6.1 mmol/l. The WSCTS guidelines suggested that both diabetics and non-diabetic patients should control their blood glucose below 10 mmol/L during cardiac surgery and early postoperative period, while the American Society of Clinical Endocrinology and the Endocrine Society (TES) recommended that the blood glucose of patients in the ICU should be maintained at 7.8–10.0 mmol/l.

7. Hypoglycemia

Currently, there is still no standard for the level of postoperative blood glucose, the amount of insulin and the treatment method. During insulin treatment, we should closely observe the changes in blood glucose, adjust the amount of insulin and strictly control blood glucose. The main adverse reaction of insulin treatment is hypoglycemia. Hypoglycemia may be an important factor leading to the deterioration or death of critically severe patients, which should be closely monitored and actively treated. Because the symptoms and signs of hypoglycemia in anaesthetized or severe patients are not easy to be detected, strict blood glucose monitoring must be carried out in order to maintain the target blood glucose floating in a small range. A large number of studies have shown that hypoglycemia is a risk factor, and defined the methods to reduce its occurrence. Many studies have reported that ICU patients are more likely to have hypoglycemia when receiving intensive insulin therapy. Recent randomized controlled trials have also shown that hypoglycemia is a significant factor affecting the prognosis and may increase the risk of mortality intensive insulin therapy. Due to the potential safety hazards associated with hypoglycemia (including increased mortality) in intensive insulin therapy, some randomized trials were terminated. Hypoglycemia is the main risk of complications in long-term intensive control therapy. Clinically, it is necessary to personalize the treatment scheme of insulin hypoglycemic therapy and reset the target blood glucose value of intensive insulin therapy.

8. Significance of perioperative glycemic control

TES recently reported that the recommended treatment regimen is that the highest blood glucose concentration of ICU patients is maintained at 110 mg/dl, and the highest blood glucose level of other inpatients is maintained at 180 mg/dl. This view has been recognized by the National Association of Anesthesiologists. The American Heart Association recently published a specific recommendation for glycemic control. Based on the reported data and the advantages and disadvantages of glycemic control, it is suggested that the target glycemic control range of patients undergoing CABG operation is 120–150 mg/dl. This range will effectively reduce the complications and mortality of intraoperative and postoperative hyperglycemia, and reduce the risk of hypoglycemia. No matter what treatment plan is applied, patients should be closely monitored and diagnosed with hyperglycemia through laboratory analysis. In particular, hyperglycemia symptoms in anaesthetized patients may be covered up. These recommended treatments may change with the progress and improvements of science and technology. For example, continuous and reliable blood glucose measurement methods can be used clinically. Based on this, strict glycemic control and minimizing the related risks are possible.

Conflict of interest

The authors declare no conflict of interest.

Author details

Cheng Luo[1], Chuan Wang[2], Xiaoyong Xie[1] and BaoShi Zheng[1*]

1 Department of Cardiac Surgery, The First Affiliated Hospital of Guangxi Medical University, Nanning, Guangxi, China

2 Department of Cardiac Surgery, Beijing Anzhen Hospital, Capital Medical University, Beijing, China

*Address all correspondence to: cnlanzhen@outlook.com

References

[1] Perez A, Levin A, Alam N. A comparison of the use of clinical-guideline-recommended antihypertensive regimens in mexican american, non-hispanic black, and non-hispanic white adults with type 2 diabetes and hypertension in the United States: NHANES 2003-2012. The Diabetes Educator. 2016;**42**(6):739-747

[2] Mancini GB, Farkouh ME, Brooks MM, Chaitman BR, Boden WE, Vlachos H, et al. Medical treatment and revascularization options in patients with type 2 diabetes and coronary disease. Journal of the American College of Cardiology. 2016;**68**(10):985-995

[3] Nyström T, Holzmann MJ, Eliasson B, Svensson AM, Kuhl J, Sartipy U. Estimated glucose disposal rate and long-term survival in type 2 diabetes after coronary artery bypass grafting. Heart and Vessels. 2017;**32**(3):269-278

[4] Ansley DM, Raedschelders K, Choi PT, Wang B, Cook RC, Chen DD. Propofol cardioprotection for on-pump aortocoronary bypass surgery in patients with type 2 diabetes mellitus (PRO-TECT II): A phase 2 randomized-controlled trial. Canadian Journal of Anaesthesia. 2016;**63**(4):442-453

[5] Klein HJ, Csordas A, Falk V, Slankamenac K, Rudiger A, Schönrath F, et al. Pancreatic stone protein predicts postoperative infection in cardiac surgery patients irrespective of cardiopulmonary bypass or surgical technique. PLoS One. 2015;**10**(3):e0120276

[6] Knapik P, Nadziakiewicz P, Urbanska E, Saucha W, Herdynska M, Zembala M. Cardiopulmonary bypass increases postoperative glycemia and insulin consumption after coronary surgery. The Annals of Thoracic Surgery. 2009;**87**(6):1859-1865

[7] Dandin E, Üstündağ ÜV, Ünal İ, Ateş-Kalkan PS, Cansız D, Beler M, et al. Stevioside ameliorates hyperglycemia and glucose intolerance, in a diet-induced obese zebrafish model, through epigenetic, oxidative stress and inflammatory regulation. Obesity Research & Clinical Practice. 2022;**16**(1):23-29. DOI: 10.1016/j.orcp.2022.01.002

[8] Meshref TS, Abd El-Aal RF, Ashry MA, Imam HM, Elden AB. Impact of stress hyperglycemia on myocardial salvage in patients with ST-Elevation myocardial infarction: Cardiac magnetic resonance study. Indian Heart Journal. 2020;**72**(5):462-465

[9] Matyal R, Sakamuri S, Huang T, Owais K, Parikh S, Khabbaz K, et al. Oxidative stress and nerve function after cardiopulmonary bypass in patients with diabetes. The Annals of Thoracic Surgery. 2014;**98**(5):1635-1643

[10] Vuori MA, Reinikainen J, Söderberg S, Bergdahl E, Jousilahti P, Tunstall-Pedoe H, et al. Diabetes status-related differences in risk factors and mediators of heart failure in the general population: results from the MORGAM/BiomarCaRE consortium. Cardiovascular Diabetology. 2021;**20**(1):195

[11] Rushani D, Tam DY, Fremes SE. Commentary: Bilateral versus single internal mammary arteries in diabetic patients undergoing coronary artery bypass grafting-is there a sweet spot? Seminars in Thoracic and Cardiovascular Surgery. 2021;**33**(2):393-394

[12] Pang PY, Lim YP, Ong KK, Chua YL, Sin YK. Young surgeon's award winner:

Long-term prognosis in patients with diabetes mellitus after coronary artery bypass grafting: A propensity-matched study. Annals of the Academy of Medicine, Singapore. 2016;**45**(3):83-90

[13] Wang C, Li P, Zhang F, Kong Q, Li J. Does bilateral internal mammary artery grafting better suit patients with diabetes? – Two different ways to explore outcomes. Circulation Journal. 2020;**84**(3):436-444

[14] Thiele RH, Hucklenbruch C, Ma JZ, Colquhoun D, Zuo Z, Nemergut EC, et al. Admission hyperglycemia is associated with poor outcome after emergent coronary bypass grafting surgery. Journal of Critical Care. 2015;**30**(6):1210-1216

[15] Klemencsics I, Lazary A, Szoverfi Z, Bozsodi A, Eltes P, Varga PP. Risk factors for surgical site infection in elective routine degenerative lumbar surgeries. The Spine Journal. 2016;**16**(11):1377-1383

[16] Lecomte P, Foubert L, Coddens J, Dewulf B, Nobels F, Casselman F, et al. Management of tight intraoperative glycemic control during off-pump coronary artery bypass surgery in diabetic and nondiabetic patients. Journal of Cardiothoracic and Vascular Anesthesia. 2011;**25**(6):937-942

[17] Schmeltz LR, DeSantis AJ, Thiyagarajan V, Schmidt K, O'Shea-Mahler E, Johnson D, et al. Reduction of surgical mortality and morbidity in diabetic patients undergoing cardiac surgery with a combined intravenous and subcutaneous insulin glucose management strategy. Diabetes Care. 2007;**30**(4):823-828

[18] Ardeshiri M, Faritus Z, Ojaghi-Haghighi Z, Bakhshandeh H, Kargar F, Aghili R. Impact of metabolic syndrome on mortality and morbidity after coronary artery bypass grafting surgery. Research in Cardiovascular Medicine. 2014;**3**(3):e20270

[19] Schwarzer M, Britton SL, Koch LG, Wisloff U, Doenst T. Low intrinsic aerobic exercise capacity and systemic insulin resistance are not associated with changes in myocardial substrate oxidation or insulin sensitivity. Basic Research in Cardiology. 2010;**105**(3):357-364

[20] Desai SP, Henry LL, Holmes SD, Hunt SL, Martin CT, Hebsur S, et al. Strict versus liberal target range for perioperative glucose in patients undergoing coronary artery bypass grafting: a prospective randomized controlled trial. The Journal of Thoracic and Cardiovascular Surgery. 2012;**143**(2):318-325

[21] Stamou SC, Nussbaum M, Carew JD, Dunn K, Skipper E, Robicsek F, et al. Hypoglycemia with intensive insulin therapy after cardiac surgery: predisposing factors and association with mortality. The Journal of Thoracic and Cardiovascular Surgeon. 2011;**142**(1):166-173

[22] Van den Berghe G, Wouters P, Weekers F, Verwaest C, Bruyninckx F, Schetz M, et al. Intensive insulin therapy in the critically ill patients. The New England Journal of Medicine. 2001;**345**:1359-1367

[23] NICE-SUGAR Study Investigators. The normoglycemia in intensive care evaluation (NICE) (ISRCTN04968275) and survival using glucose algorithm regulation (SUGAR) Study: development, design and conduct of an international multi-center, open label, randomized controlled trial of two target ranges for glycemic control in intensive care unit patients. American Journal of Respiratory and Critical Care Medicine. 2005;**172**:1358-1359

Section 2

Various Techniques of Coronary Artery Bypass Grafting

Chapter 4

Off-Pump Coronary Artery Bypass (OPCAB), the New Conventional Coronary Artery Bypass (CCAB) Technique

Murali P. Vettath, Arunachalam Vellachamy Kannan, Ganagadharan Nitin, Siddegowda Nagaraju Gururkirana, Koroth Smera, Raman Gopalakrishnan and A.K. Baburajan

Abstract

Coronary artery bypass grafting (CABG), has evolved over the last twenty-five years. Having pioneered this evolution for the last two decades and more, we have moved from an on-pump surgical unit to a completely off-pump surgical unit. This on-pump surgery was in vogue for the past six decades. This was labeled the Conventional CABG (CCAB). We have over the last two decades made off-pump coronary artery bypass (OPCAB) the new CCAB. To make this a reality, we had to invent, innovate, fabricate and modify techniques and technology, so as to make ourselves comfortable to perform all our CABGs without the use of the Heart-lung machine (HLM). We have over the last twenty years performed more than five thousand OPCAB surgeries in this city alone, with a mortality of less than 1%.

In this chapter, we would like to elucidate how one could master this technique of performing OPCAB in all patients who need CABG.

Keywords: CABG, CCAB, OPCAB

1. Introduction

Since 1967, when Rene Favalaro performed the first CABG, using saphenous vein graft (SVG) on an arrested heart [1], at Cleveland clinic, till 1985, when Buffallo [2] and Bennetti [3], published their OPCAB report, on-pump CABG was considered the CCAB. In fact, their publication kindled the fire to develop OPCAB in many surgeons around the world.

Conventional CABG was the gold standard all over the world for the last five decades, probably even now in most of countries. As going on Cardiopulmonary bypass (CPB), stopping the heart and performing the anastomosis on a bloodless and motionless heart was quite a reproducible surgical technique by most of coronary surgeons around the world. This was performed by connecting the heart to the heart-lung machine, using a cross-clamp on the aorta, and giving Cardioplegia (CP), in the root of the aorta (antegrade CP), or into the coronary sinus (retrograde CP). Then the distal coronary anastomosis was performed in a bloodless and motionless heart. Here, only surgical anastomosis was to be mastered. This became very popular, and this became the CCAB. But with the advent of coronary angioplasty and stenting and the arrival of drug-eluting stents, the number of patients having complications on the HLM started to surface. Basically, the inherent effects of the pump, the inflammatory response, and the development of stroke in the diseased aorta, where cannulations had to be done, and where the cross-clamp had to be used, all became dreaded complications of CABG, and so the number of patients coming for CABG reduced. Cardiologists became the gatekeepers, and so it was time for a change to happen. Hence, with the idea of OPCAB mooted by the South American duo, we in the east started working on how to perform CABG without the use of HLM.

Then in the late 1990s in Utrecht, Netherland, OCTOPUS, the stabilizer was developed, which paved the way for OPCAB to become a reality [4].

2. Anesthetic modifications for OPCAB

Unlike in on-pump CABG, in OPCAB we had to modify our anesthetic technique, to maintain adequate hemodynamics all through surgery. We in fact stop beta blockers on the day of surgery. The main difference between on-pump and off-pump surgery is that in on-pump if the patient crashes during induction, we can go on CPB and revive the patient. We routinely use an internal jugular four-lumen cannula and a radial and femoral arterial line before starting surgery. The femoral arterial line is used to insert the IABP when needed. In OPCAB the anesthetist has to be very vigilant to make sure we do not drop the pressures below a mean of 75 mm of mercury (Hg), all through the procedure. The mean pressure has to be maintained by using small doses of vasopressors, as and when required. Especially when the heart is positioned. It's with a combination of table movement and the use of these vasopressors judiciously, that the anesthetist maintains hemodynamics all through the procedure. The anesthesia is usually maintained by a combination of Fentanyl, Midazolam, Dexmedetomedine, and muscle relaxant cisatracurium. All coronary patients have an infusion of Lasix, during surgery. Routinely our patients are ventilated postoperatively overnight. Once stable, they are weaned and extubated in the morning.

3. OPCAB and its progression

In the nineties, surgeons including us were trying our hand at stabilizing the square centimeter of myocardium that needed to be grafted, using all sorts of instrumentation, which obviously was not reproducible. Then we used to use injection of Adenosine to stop the heartbeat during the crucial stich on the heel and the toes and restart the heart using pacing wires, etc. Again this technique did not work too.

Only after the Octopus stabilizers came, we could start performing OPCABs routinely. The intracoronary shunts were a very important invention that paved the way for routine use of OPCABs as a procedure of choice.

Initially, our thought was to reduce the heartbeats so that we would have less movement of the heart and we had more time to place our sutures properly. But then we noticed that after using too much of beta blockers, we needed inotropes to get the heart going in the post-operative period. This we had to tackle by stopping these beta blockers on the day of surgery. As we developed a technique of using Injection Atropine to increase the heart rate, then slowing it down, which improved our hemodynamics, and our stabilizers would do their job by mechanically stopping the movement. This technique was useful for all our anterior wall grafting.

4. Grafting the lateral wall vessels

Then came the issue of grafting the lateral and posterior wall vessels. So, for the lateral wall vessels, we routinely open the right pleura and then cut the pericardium down to the Inferior vena cava (IVC). This allows the right heart to fall into the right chest, while the heart is lifted and verticalized to visualize the lateral wall vessels. Earlier we used the Positioners to lift the apex and tilt the heart, but off late, with experience, we use a deep pericardial stitch [5] to lift the heart up to get easy access to the lateral wall. By doing so the hemodynamics are maintained. Then the stabilizer is placed at the respective positions and the grafting progressed.

5. Grafting the posterior wall vessels

Positioning is important for grafting all these vessels. For the posterior wall, the table is lifted up, and then the head end is dropped as in Trendelenburg position.

If the heart flops too much to the right pleura, then a pericardial stay is used on the detached right pleura to keep the heart vertical. Wet sponges are used to position the heart in the lateral side. Now with the heart positioned, the stabilizer is used to stabilize either the PDA or the PLV as planned. And the grafting progressed as usual.

If the right coronary artery (RCA) is to be grafted, we use a stabilizer with suction pods so that that area to be grafted on the RCA is stabilized and lifted up a bit. So, to say, that, we don't use suction on the pods either for the LAD or the circumflex coronary artery grafts. usually.

For grafting the RCA, we usually use 2 snares of 5.0 prolene suture, one proximal and one distal to the proposed site of the coronary incision. Once the snares are placed, the coronary opening is made and the shunt inserted, then the snares are released, and the grafting is performed as usual. For RCA grafts, the pacing wires are kept ready in case the heart slow.

6. Top-end anastomosis

Usually, the top-end of the vein grafts are performed using a side clamp on the aorta. But in the case of patients with disease aorta, applying a side clamp will lead to dispersing the plaques into the cerebral vessels and causing the stroke. Hence, in patients with the diseased aorta, we had invented our own top-end anastomosing device, the Vettaths anastomotic obturator (VAO) [6]. This has been patented and has been extensively used by us to perform the top end of more than five hundred patients. This has been published in different journals [7]. This is quite useful and does not increase the cost of surgery.

Coming to the top-end anastomosis technique, when we have a patient with chronic renal failure, either on dialysis or with just elevated renal function, OPCAB is more excellent than going on the pump. In such patients, we try and avoid hypotension as much as possible. In case we need to avoid the hypotension completely, then we use the VAO, where we can still maintain the systolic pressure above 100 mm of Hg. But if the creatinine is below 2 mg/dl, and the ascending aorta is not diseased, then when we use a side clamp, we maintain the systolic pressure between 85 and 90 and perform only one top end of the vein graft, and the other is hooked on to this vein graft as a piggyback. This is such that the mean pressure is attained between, 75 and 80 mm of Hg all the time.

Vettath's technique of mammary patch for diffusely disease LAD without endarterectomy [8].

This is yet another of our innovative technique, in patients who present with diffuse CAD in young age and are deemed inoperable in most centers and are ischemic. We have also published this technique in many journals and are readily available online [8]. The videos are also available in YouTube. The good thing about these techniques are that these patients are able to live a comfortable life without any symptoms. This is a common disease seen in the youth in this part of the world, where stenting is not possible.

7. Role of intra-aortic balloon pump (IABP)

Intra-aortic balloon pump is the most accessible left ventricular assist device that has been in use since its development by Christenson [9, 10]. He had proposed to use the IABP postoperatively initially and later proposed to use it even preoperatively, to stabilize the heart and give a rest to the myocardium, by increasing the coronary flow.

In 2016 [11] we published an article explaining our modification of the role of IABP in OPCAB, which we are still practicing, till date. We have not used IABP, since the day before surgery so far. When the patient is very ischemic with severe ST changes and with hemodynamic instability and complaining of chest pain before induction, we have inserted the IABP, through the Femoral arterial line, which we use to monitor the arterial pressure routinely. This is inflated and this augments the coronary perfusion, thereby preventing ischemia. We give 5000IU of injection heparin to insert this under local anesthesia. Though this is a rare occurrence, we have had to do this in spite of our excellent anesthesia techniques, which we have also standardized over the last two decades.

Most of the time we just insert the femoral arterial line after induction, even in patients with tight left main stenosis, if the patient is hemodynamically stable during induction and is able to maintain a mean blood pressure above 75 mm of mercury(Hg). Hence the use of IABP comes mostly while grafting the lateral wall vessels, that too only in big ischemic obtuse marginal with tight stenosis, proximally and having a dynamic mitral regurgitation noticed in echo preoperatively.

Our grafting techniques are pretty standard, as we first take down the LIMA, skeletonized (https://www.youtube.com/watch?v=m7mYWLQsDAE). Then Heparin is given and flow assessed. The radial artery is used for circumflex vessels sometimes. The long saphenous vein is taken as a skip technique, taking care not to cause intimal injury.

Once the LIMA is anastomosed to the LAD, most of the time patient becomes stable. We are then able to lift the heart and position it to expose the lateral wall, using the stitch in the deep pericardial well. If the pulmonary artery pressure goes up by looking at it or we feel that the heart has started distending and is slowing down, we immediately take the packs out and release the LIMA stitch and increase the heart rate after lifting the head end up, like an anti-Trendelenburg position. This is exactly what the patient would do in his bed when he develops chest pain. Hereby, the left ventricular end-diastolic pressure comes down and reduces the sub-endocardial ischemia. Now the heart looks better. If this is not working, we insert the IABP, without the sheath and inflate it and keep it going till the distal anastomosis of the circumflex vessels are done. We then go in and perform the top end anastomosis, either using a side clamp or the VAO, whichever is found necessary. While performing the top end anastomosis, the IABP is usually in a standby position. Usually, after the top end is performed and the side clamp removed the heart jumps back to normal hemodynamics, and we are able to perform the usual PDA anastomosis even without the IABP. Hence after all the grafting is done, we reverse the Heparin with protamine. After 5 minutes of Heparin reversal, we are usually able to remove the IABP, after inserting another femoral arterial line in the opposite side. This technique has been useful in the sense that we have avoided the conversion on to the HLM in most of the patients. So, to say, over the last 14 years, we had to go on to the heart-lung machine only once. That too, when the patient developed uncontrollable arrhythmia. This patient ended up having the IABP being taken to the cardiac surgical ICU with the patient. Other than this all the IABPs if used in the operation theatre are removed in the OT itself.

From	To	No. of OPCAB	Conversion	IABP	Mortality
Jul-02	Dec-02	47	0	0	0
Jan-03	Dec-03	177	12	0	0
Jan-04	Dec-04	238	6	0	1
Jan-05	Dec-05	299	0	0	3
Jan-06	Dec-06	284	0	4	5
Jan-07	Dec-07	260	1	8	0
Jan-08	Dec-08	225	0	11	2
Jan-09	Dec-09	280	0	8	0
Jan-10	Dec-10	358	0	22	0
Jan-11	Dec-11	413	0	24	0
Jan-12	Dec-12	425	0	23	2
Jan-13	Dec-13	429	0	18	2
Jan-14	Dec-14	312	0	6	3
Jan-15	Dec-15	317	0	6	2
Jan-16	Dec-16	228	0	11	3
Jan-17	Dec-17	109	0	0	0
Jan-18	Dec-18	196	0	0	0
Jan-19	Dec-19	212	1	7	3
Jan-20	Dec-20	128	0	2	2
Jan-21	Dec-21	159	0	1	3
7/4/2002	12/31/2021	5096	20 (0.39%)	151 (2.96%)	31 (0.60%)

This is our modification of IABP, which we have been following. (Chart) [11].

8. Training to be an OPCAB surgeon

Any cardiac surgeon who is interested in becoming an off-pump surgeon, has to first become good on-pump surgeon, and must have an excellent result on-pump, only then should he venture to perform OPCAB.

A perfect coronary anastomosis is the gold standard of CABG. How it's achieved is the prerogative of the surgeon. And depends upon his skill and mindset. Once he is able to dissect a perfect Internal mammary artery, first left and next the right, and to harvest the radial artery and the saphenous veins in that order, and then perform the anastomosis with them, on the pump, only then should he go off-pump.

It is important for the surgeon to visit a good OPCAB center and spend some time there to see how they do it and then try to transfer the technique to his practice.

We started this journey 20 years ago and it took us more than five hundred OPCABs to standardize our technique. When we started off, we were prepared for all eventualities, like going back on pump, whenever we felt it was not safe, or when hemodynamics became bad. Our technique has been elaborated in previous chapters we have published [12].

We had developed our own OPCAB stabilizer, the simple Indian-made stabilizer (SIMS), which has been sent for patenting in 2015. The video link of OPCAB using SIMS in youTube- https://www.youtube.com/playlist?list=PLmvb6npEfabinhlatq8IY LBz8WlHo8bu1

We have been routinely using it for all our surgeries over the last thousand five hundred cases. For the last hundred-odd cases. This stabilizer is shown in **Figure 1** below.

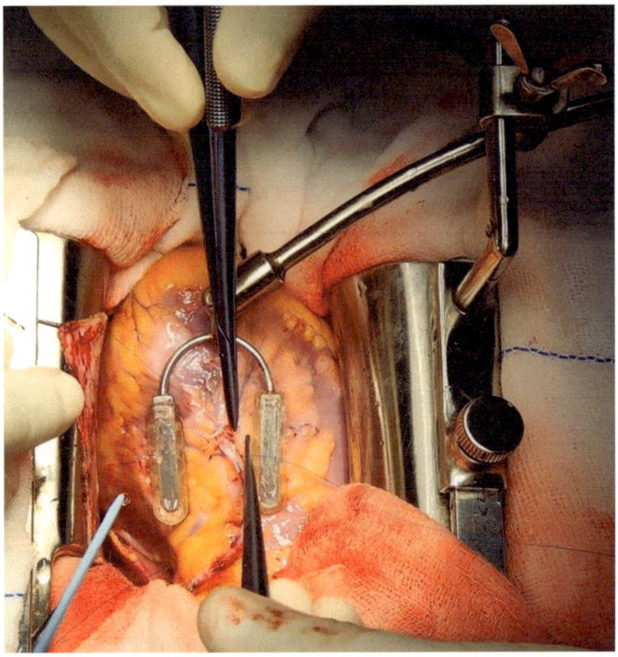

Figure 1.
Shows SIMS with the new Pods.

We started off with first retaining the aortic cannula alone, then when we became confident, that was out as well. And gradually went on and on, and after 20 years and 5000 odd cases, we have had to convert to the heart-lung machine in only one patient in the last 14 years. The reason was the patient developed uncontrolled arrhythmia and could not stabilize with IABP.

9. Future of OPCAB

Minimally invasive and Robotic OPCABs would be the future of coronary revascularization. Though we have performed quite a few of them in this center itself, with multiple grafts, the risk and results are not that as we have in midline sternotomy. Hence, we have set it aside for single or maximum double grafts. We have also developed our own stabilizer for minimally invasive OPCAB too (**Figure 2**).

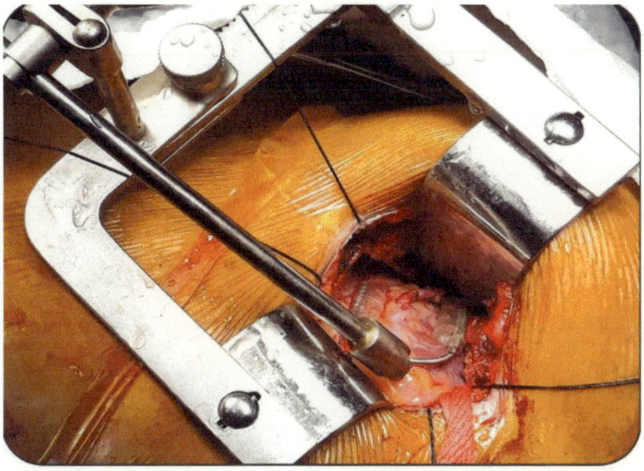

Figure 2.
Shows the modified SIMS for MICS OPCAB.

Author details

Murali P. Vettath[1*], Arunachalam Vellachamy Kannan[2], Ganagadharan Nitin[3], Siddegowda Nagaraju Gururkirana[1], Koroth Smera[2], Raman Gopalakrishnan[2] and A.K. Baburajan[1]

1 Department of Cardiac Surgery, Meitra Hospital, Kozhikode, Kerala, India

2 Department of Cardiac Anaesthesia, Meitra Hospital, Kozhikode, Kerala, India

3 Department of Anaesthesia, Meitra Hospital, Kozhikode, Kerala, India

*Address all correspondence to: murali.vettath@gmail.com

References

[1] Favaloro RG. Saphenous vein graft in the surgical treatment of coronary artery disease. Thoracic Cardiovascular Surgery. 1968;**58**:178-185

[2] Buffolo E, Andrade JCS, Succi JE, et al. Direct myocardial revascularization without cardiopulmonary bypass. Thoracic Cardiovascular Surgery. 1985;**33**:26-29

[3] Benetti FJ. Direct coronary surgery with saphenous vein bypass without either cardiopulmonary bypass or cardiac arrest. Journal of Cardiovascular Surgery. 1985;**26**:217-222

[4] Borst C, Jansen EW, Tulleken CA, et al. Coronary artery bypass grafting without cardiopulmonary bypass and without interruption of native coronary flow using a novel anastomosis site restraining device ("Octopus"). Journal of the American College Cardiology. 1996;**27**:1356-1364

[5] Bergsland J, Karamanoukian HL, Soltoski PR, Salerno TA. "Single Suture" for circumflex exposure in OffPump coronary artery bypass grafting. Annals of the Thoracic Surgery. 1999;**68**:1428-1430

[6] Vettath MP. Vettath's anastomotic obturator: A simple proximal anastomotic device. The Heart Surgery Forum. 2003;**6**:366-368. Available from: www.hsforum.com/vol6/issue5/2003-73305.html pp-366-368

[7] Murali VP. Vettath's anastamotic obturator—Our experience of 269 proximal anastamosis. Heart Lung and Circulation. 2004;**13**:288-290

[8] Prabhu AD, Thazhkuni IE, Rajendran S, et al. Mammary patch reconstruction of left anterior descending coronary artery. Asian Cardiovascular & Thoracic Annals. 2008a;**16**:313-317

[9] Christenson JT, Simonet F, Badel P, Schmuziger M. Evaluation of preoperative intra-aortic balloon pump support in high risk coronary patients. European Journal of Cardiothoracic Surgery. 1997;**11**:1097-1103

[10] Christenson J, Simonet F, Badel P, Schmuziger M. Optimal timing of preoperative intraaortic balloon pump support in high-risk coronary patients. Annals of the Thoracic Surgery. 1999;**68**:934-939

[11] Vettath MP et al. Role of intra-aortic balloon pump in off pump coronary artery bypass—A Vettath modification. World Journal of Cardiovascular Diseases. 2016;**6**:188-195

[12] Vettath MP, Vellachamy KA, Ganagadharan N, Ravisankar M, Koroth S, Gopalakrishnan Raman G. Revascularisation strategies in OPCAB (Off Pump Coronary Artery Bypass). DOI: 10.5772/intechopen.88102f 12–PP-91-104

Chapter 5

Coronary-Coronary Bypass Grafting

Vladlen Bazylev, Dmitry Tungusov and Artur Mikulyak

Abstract

This work is devoted to the original method of myocardial revascularization—coronary-coronary bypass grafting. Coronary artery bypass grafting can be considered as an independent method in an exceptional case or as an addition to the standard coronary artery bypass grafting technique. This paper presents the technique for performing CCBG, as well as the early and long-term results of the main studies. Attention is also paid to the advantages and disadvantages of this method from the standpoint of physiology and physics.

Keywords: coronary artery bypass graft surgery, myocardial revascularization

1. Introduction

"Difficulties are meant to rouse, not discourage."
William Ellery Channing

Coronary artery bypass grafting (CABG) with the use of saphenous vein grafts (SVG) and the left internal thoracic artery (ITA) is the standard of myocardial revascularization for many cardiac surgeons. But in everyday practice, the course of the surgery can change dramatically. Calcification of aortic root and ascending aorta, grafts limitation and lesion of subclavian artery are leading to a search for alternative sources of blood supply. One of those alternatives is the coronary artery itself. In coronary-coronary bypass grafting (CCBG), proximal and distal anastomoses are performed between one or more coronary arteries with the use of different conduits.

2. History of coronary-coronary bypass grafting and its reported outcomes

In the case of coronary-coronary bypass grafting, proximal and distal anastomoses are formed between different coronary arteries or segments of the same coronary artery. This technique requires a native proximal coronary artery to provide adequate distal flow. The idea of using the proximal portion of the coronary artery as an alternative source of blood supply came to several researchers almost simultaneously. In 1987, CCBG was described by Biglioli and colleagues [1]. The authors present their experience with coronary-coronary bypass grafting. The most usual site of proximal implantation for CCBG in this series was the origin of the RCA. According to Biglioli et al., this technique takes advantage of physiological position of the right coronary artery ostium: the filling of the graft and of the coronary circulation is assisted by several factors promoting the physiological diastolic coronary artery blood flow.

In the same 1987 Nishida et al. in a 62-year-old man used the proximal part of coronary artery to bypass distal vessels when other conventional grafting techniques are not possible [2]. In this patient, a saphenous vein graft was not possible to use, for this reason, the free right internal thoracic artery was used for grafting the right coronary artery. The proximal anastomosis was performed to RCA and distal one to posterior descending artery. The postoperative period of the patient and recovery progressed without any complications. Patient was discharged with no angina. Three months after bypass surgery, the coronary angiography was performed and that revealed patency of the coronary-coronary bypass graft.

Rowland et al, in 1987 also reported on the possibility of coronary-coronary bypass grafting in an emergency situation [3]. In one case this technique was performed on a 75-year-old man with significant chronic obstructive pulmonary disease (COPD), diabetes mellitus and left below-knee amputation. This patient was admitted with unstable angina. The coronary angiography revealed the circumflex artery with 99% proximal stenosis and two large, nondiseased distal obtuse marginal branches (OM). The left anterior descending (LAD) had a 70% proximal stenosis, and the right coronary artery showed a 50% lesion at the middle part. Distal runoff was unaffected. Intraoperatively the aortic arch and ascending aorta were found calcified for cannulation or proximal anastomosis excluding the small area of aorta, next to the ostium of right coronary artery, that was found to be suitable for cross-clamping. The cardiopulmonary bypass was established via peripheral cannulation. The proximal part of right coronary artery was separated and was found intact. CCBG was performed between proximal part of right coronary artery, obtuse marginal arteries and left anterior descending artery. The postoperative period was complicated by development of the left hemispheric stroke, kidney and hepatic failure, arrhythmias and prolonged ventilation and pneumonia as a result. The patient died two months postoperatively of noncardiac complications.

In the second case, CCBG was performed on a 59-year-old woman who had phlebectomy in anamnesis. Patient was admitted with an inferior myocardial infarction. The coronary angiography showed the right coronary artery with 40% proximal stenosis with a good distal runoff, and the 99% proximal of circumflex artery with good distal runoff. LAD had 85% stenosis located between the first and second diagonal arteries with a good distal runoff. Intraoperatively, only a short saphenous vein was available for harvesting. The left internal thoracic artery was not long enough for grafting the circumflex system. For complete revascularization bifurcated saphenous vein was used for coronary-coronary bypass grafting. Anastomoses were performed between the first diagonal artery, circumflex artery, left anterior descending artery and intact second diagonal branch. The postoperative course was uneventful, and four months later, the patient completed treadmill testing with no chest pain and no ischemic changes in ECG.

Thus, three independent researchers at almost the same time proposed a solution to one of the most difficult problems in coronary surgery. Further references to coronary-coronary bypass surgery were episodic. Basically, these are case descriptions using different conduits, as well as different observation periods.

Erdil N. et al. reported a CCBG in a 74-year-old man with a calcified ascending aorta [4]. Anastomoses were performed between proximal and distal parts of right coronary artery with a saphenous vein graft, while the left internal thoracic artery was anastomosed to the left anterior descending artery. Surgery was performed without cardiopulmonary bypass. The patient survived without negative evidence. Angiography showed graft patency one year after revascularization. Possibility of coronary-coronary bypasses grafting off-pump in patients with extensive atherosclerotic aorta was also described by Yalcikaya A. et al. and Wan L.F. et al [5].

Marisalco G. described the case of functioning of a coronary-coronary graft for 19 years. CCBG was performed to minimize manipulation of a porcelain ascending aorta. Sequential coronary-coronary bypass grafts had been performed using a saphenous vein graft from the proximal right coronary artery to the left anterior descending artery and the obtuse marginal branch [6].

Denis B. in 1995 used the radial artery for coronary-coronary bypass grafting. He performed anastomosis between proximal and terminal parts of the RCA. The postoperative course was uneventful. A control coronary angiogram performed on day 6 showed an excellent result with a good match of the RA graft and the distal RCA [7].

However, among the description of single cases, some researchers analyzed a series of such surgeries. Nottin R. et al. reported about 143 patients underwent myocardial revascularization with one (138 patients) or two (5 patients) coronary-coronary bypass grafts in addition to other bypass grafts, for a total of 463 distal anastomoses (mean 3.2 ± 0.6 per patient) [8]. In this study the coronary-coronary

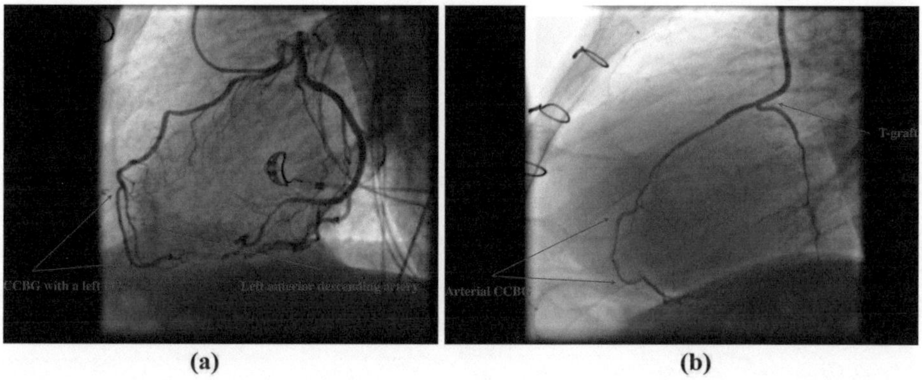

Figure 1.
Angiography of coronary-coronary bypasses graft. (a) Isolated CCBG of the left anterior descending artery. (b) Simultaneous CCBG and composite arterial grafting.

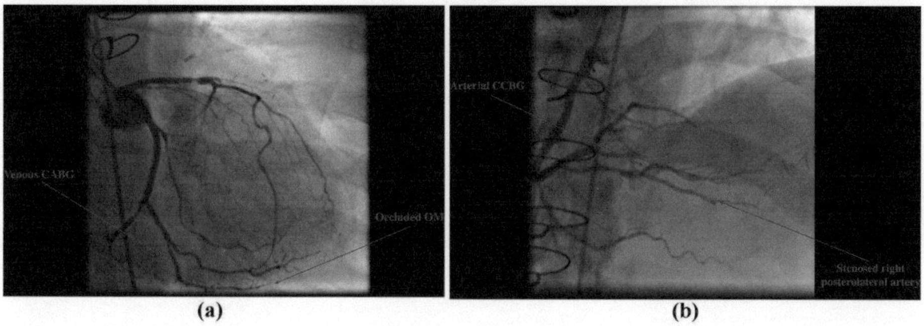

Figure 2.
Angiography of coronary-coronary bypasses graft. (a) Saphenous vein for the circumflex/branches of the circumflex. (b) Internal thoracic artery for right coronary–posterior descending/right posterolateral artery.

bypass grafts were chosen for the following reasons: arterial conduit-sparing procedure, inadequate length for in situ graft, calcified ascending aorta and stenosed or occluded subclavian arteries. For complete revascularization, the authors used both arterial and venous conduits. Coronary-coronary bypass grafts were performed for right, circumflex and anterior descending coronary arteries. Three patients (2%) died of myocardial infarction. Early postoperative angiography showed a patency rate of 98.6% (72/73). During the mean follow-up of 34.6–20.8 months,

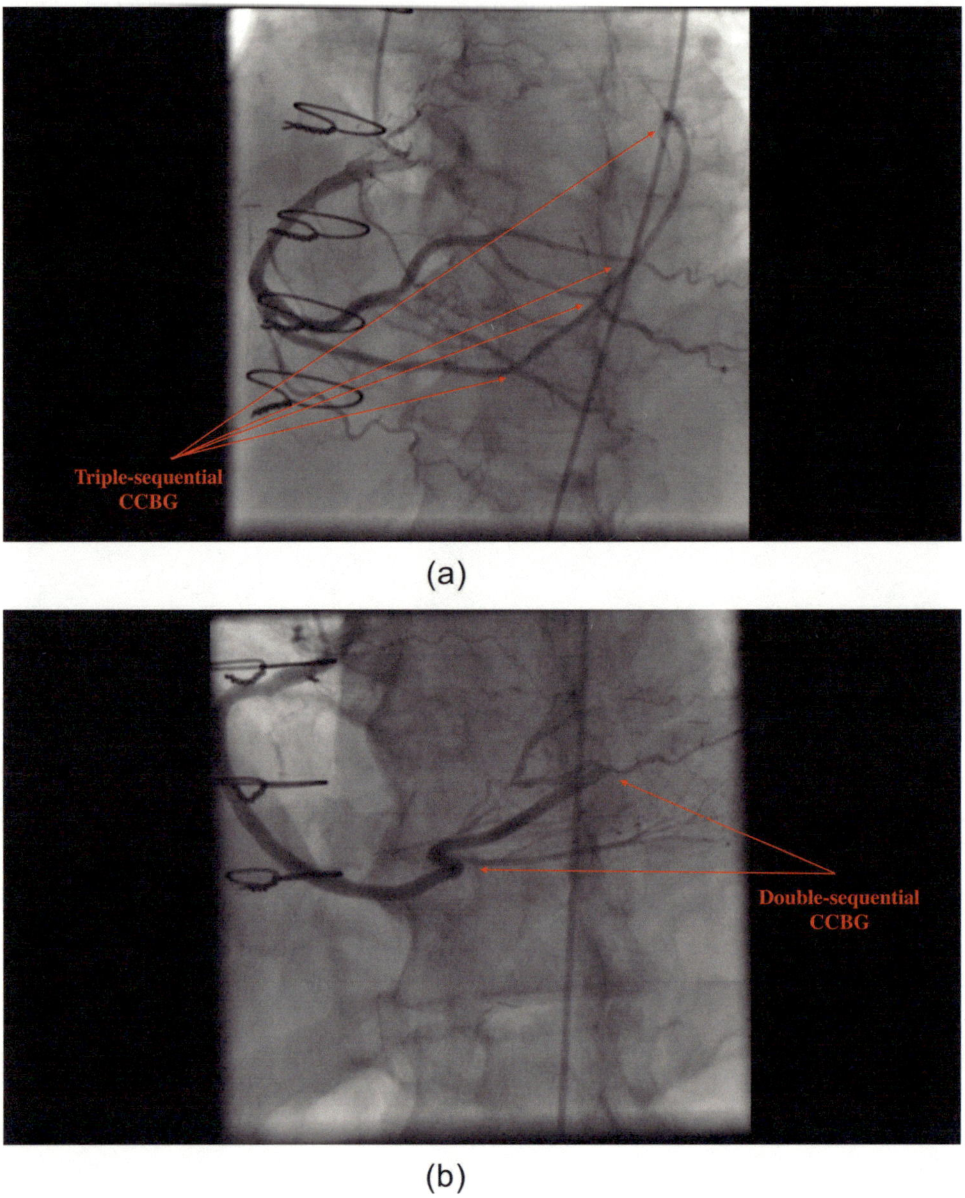

Figure 3.
Angiography of coronary-coronary bypasses graft. (a) Internal thoracic artery for right coronary–posterior descending/right posterolateral artery. (b) Saphenous vein for right coronary–right coronary/posterior descending/right posterolateral artery.

two patients died and two underwent reoperation. In this study, the authors did not provide long-term angiographic data. However, researchers of Federal Center for Cardiovascular Surgery (Penza) carried out an angiographic controlled study of the long-term results of CCBG. This study enrolled 95 patients. All patients underwent angiographic assessment of the coronary bypass grafts in the long-term follow-up period. The observation period was up to 123 months (mean 64.5 ± 24.4 months) [9].

Angiography in different types of CCBG is presented above. **Figure 1A** shows coronary-coronary bypass grafting of the distal left anterior descending artery with a left ITA segment, while the left ITA in situ was used to bypass obtuse marginal branch. In **Figure 1B**, the proximal part of the left anterior descending artery was grafted with a T-graft and the distal part was revascularized by CCBG. In a number of cases, CCBG was performed when the lesion of coronary artery was too distal for using internal thoracic artery in situ. To avoid the tension of the conduits CCBGs were used for grafting the distal parts of coronary arteries.

CCBG also allowed multiple arterial revascularizations while it was possible to save the ITA. Sometimes, the proximity of an occluded or stenosed coronary artery to a native patent coronary artery is predisposed to CCBG (**Figure 2A** and **B**).

In most cases, linear grafting was performed. However, there were 6 cases of sequential shunting: 3 cases of double (**Figure 3B**) and 3 cases of triple-sequential grafting (**Figure 3A**).

In a number of cases, CCBG was performed when it was impossible to form a proximal anastomosis with the aorta (limited length of conduit, calcification of the ascending aorta, etc.).

The early postoperative period was uneventful for all patients. In none of the cases, ischemic electrocardiogram changes or an increase in cardiac biomarkers were observed. No operative or hospital mortality occurred. The mean intensive care unit stay was 2±1.5 days and hospital stay was 9±4.5 days.

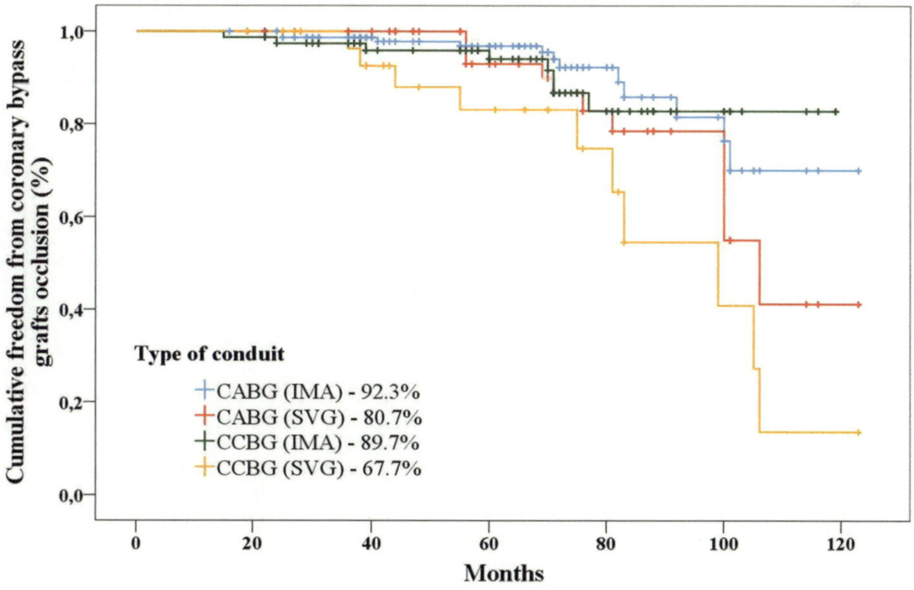

Figure 4.
Cumulative freedom from coronary bypass graft occlusion (Kaplan-Meier analysis). CABG: coronary artery bypass grafting; CCBG: coronary-coronary bypass grafting; ITA: internal thoracic artery; and SVG: saphenous vein graft.

Researchers assessed the efficacy and safety of CCBG added to the conventional technique of myocardial revascularization. In total 156 arterial, 67 venous and 109 coronary-coronary grafts were assessed. Coronary angiography was performed after recurrence of clinic of chest pain. According to the results, 12 (7.6%) arterial and 11 (19.3%) venous conduits were occluded, as well as 8 (10.3%) arterial and 10 (31.3%) venous coronary-coronary grafts. Kaplan-Meier analysis demonstrated differences in the occlusion of conduit (**Figure 4**).

According to results of research, the probability of occlusion of venous CCBG was significantly higher than that of arterial coronary-coronary grafts and ITA (log rank p ¼ 0.001 and 0.008, respectively) [9].

3. Operative technique of CCBG

In all described cases, revascularization was performed via median sternotomy. There are 3 techniques for the arterial grafts harvesting:

- pedicled, including internal thoracic veins, perivascular adipose, muscle and fascia;
- semiskeletonized, including only internal thoracic veins;
- skeletonized, only the internal thoracic artery.

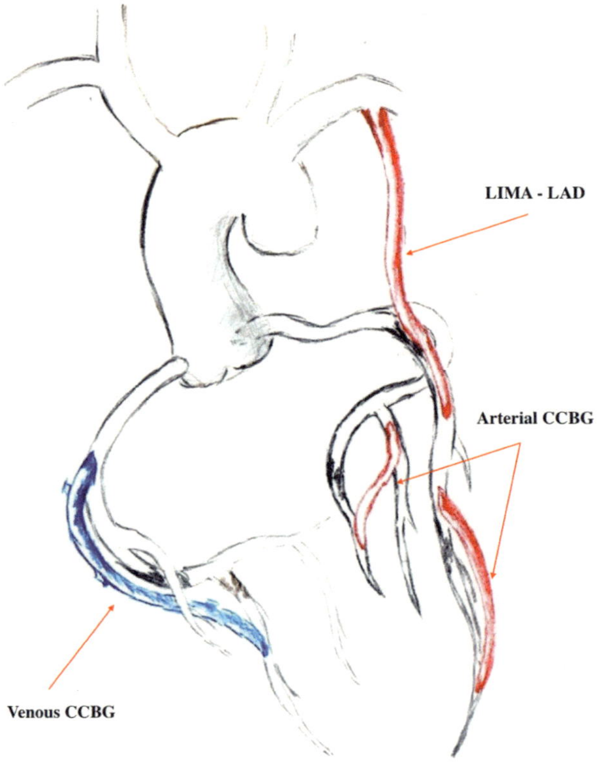

Figure 5.
The scheme of revascularization for the left and right coronary artery.

It should be noted that pedicled and semiskeletonized harvesting of ITAs significantly reduces the length of the arterial conduit. In the case of a lack of transplants, the situation will worsen much. Systemic hypo-coagulation was achieved by infusion of unfractionated heparin (calculated dose 3 mg/kg^{-1}).

The most usual site of proximal implantation for CCBG was the proximal part of the RCA [7, 10]. According to many authors, the initial segment of the RCA was often free of atherosclerosis and adequate diameter and thickness of this vessel also allowed a satisfactory congruence of the anastomosis with the graft. Other sites of proximal implantation are also possible. Bazylev V. and Nottin R. reported about using of branches of circumflex artery and LAD. CCBG was performed either between two segments of the same coronary artery or between its branches, generally the RCA or Cx. The **Figure** 5 shows the scheme of complete myocardial revascularization with the use of CCBG technique.

4. Potential advantages and disadvantages of CCBG

Initially, coronary-coronary bypass grafts were described as an alternative method of myocardial revascularization in patients with a limited number of conduits suitable for grafting and/or severe calcification of the ascending aorta and its branches. In most cases, the use of this technique has been accidental and forced. Nevertheless, available data demonstrate the possibility of using coronary-coronary bypass grafting as an isolated intervention or as an addition to the standard CABG [11]. Information on the use of CCBG is limited, but the accumulated experience indicates patency of these grafts for decades.

Such long-term efficiency has its own physiological preconditions. Many authors have shown the hemodynamic advantages of coronary-coronary bypass grafts over saphenous vein grafted to the ascending aorta [12]. Proximal anastomoses formed with the coronary artery itself provide a diastolic character to the blood flow and a less pronounced Venturi effect. According to the law of Bernoulli-Venturi, the difference in diameter is accompanied by a change in speed and pressure in places of vessel recalibration. Thus, the velocity of the blood passing through a constricted area will increase and its static pressure will decrease. Exactly in the place of diameter change the generated turbulent flow affects the state of the endothelium.

Similar conclusions can be reached if we consider the hemodynamic changes in the grafts from the viewpoint of wall share stress alteration. The pathophysiological significance of wall shear stress has been described not so long ago. Wall share stress is directly proportional to the average velocity of blood flow and inversely proportional to the inner radius of the vessel. Low values of these parameters allow accelerating the development of atherosclerotic plaques with thickening of the intima and fibromuscular dysplasia and platelet aggregation [13]. For example, in the study of Bazylev V. et al. the frequency of occluded venous coronary-coronary bypass grafts was higher than arterial ones: 8 (10.3%) vs. 10 (31.3%). One of the indirect reasons for the failure of venous coronary-coronary bypass grafts in the long-term period could be a larger diameter of the venous transplants, and as a result, a more pronounced hemodynamic effect on the vascular wall.

One of the problems of coronary-coronary bypass grafting can be the blood flow discreditation of the donor artery. Nottin and colleagues described their early postoperative results where 3 patients died from recurrent myocardial infarction. However, the mean aortic crossclamp time and the average number of distal anastomoses in this study were 83±27 min and 3.23±0.67, respectively. Results of Bazylev and colleagues show the uneventful early postoperative period in both groups of patients. In no case, ischemic electrocardiogram changes or an increase in cardiac biomarkers were observed. The reason for this may lie in the shorter period of myocardial ischemia but comparable number of distal anastomoses (61±42 min and 3,4±1,19, respectively).

Another problem of CCBG could be the progression of atherosclerosis in the region of proximal anastomosis. Bruschke and colleagues explored the progression of atherosclerosis in the RCA in 256 patients who were not operated on. Researchers found that the proximal and middle parts of the right coronary artery were most addicted to the progression of atherosclerosis, while no progression of atherosclerosis in the ostium and first segment (before the conus branch) was observed [14].

The choice of conduit for CCBG also remains controversial. Many studies have shown that the patency of CABG mostly depends on the type of conduit used. This statement is true for CCBG also. Patency of coronary-coronary bypass grafts does not depend on the progression of atherosclerosis in the donor coronary artery but depends on the type of conduit used. Extrapolating the results of using the ITA in situ, many researchers believe that the ITA is the best conduit for this procedure. Korkmaz et al. and Nishida et al. believed that even as a coronary-coronary graft, the internal thoracic artery has a number of advantages such as resistance to atherosclerosis due to prostacyclin secretion, and a low tendency to vasospasm compared to radial artery [2, 15]. Nevertheless, the effectiveness of SVG has also been described. Bazylev V. and collogues used both arterial and venous transplants, but it is difficult to confirm the superiority or disadvantages of any graft because this study was a retrospective and single-centre based on a relatively small number of observations. The authors were not taking into account the quality of the grafts (diameter, possible damage, etc.). The overall patency rates may be overestimated because some patients did not have angiograms for several reasons also. However, it was found that the patency of venous CCBG was lower than that of arterial CCBG. It can be assumed that venous coronary-coronary bypass grafts, as well as CABG, obey the same laws. Thus, neointimal hyperplasia, appearance and progression of atherosclerosis in the venous transplants may be manifestations of the hemodynamic qualities described earlier.

Further study of CCBG is warranted and will improve the results of coronary bypass surgery.

5. Conclusion

Arterial CCBG represents an alternative technique that allows complete myocardial revascularization.

Conflict of interest

The authors declare no conflict of interest.

Author details

Vladlen Bazylev, Dmitry Tungusov and Artur Mikulyak*
Federal State Budgetary Institution “Federal Center for Cardiovascular Surgery” of the Ministry of Health of the Russian Federation, Penza, Russia

*Address all correspondence to: mikulyak.artur@gmail.com

References

[1] Biglioli P, Almanni F, Antona S, Sala A, Susini G. Coronary-coronary bypass: theoretical basis and techniques. The Journal of Cardiovascular Surgery. 1987;**28**:333-335

[2] Nishida H, Grooters RK, Endo M, et al. Flow study of coronary-coronary bypass grafting. Cardiovascular Surgery. 1993;**1**:296-299

[3] Rowland PE, Grooters RK. Coronary-coronary artery bypass: An alternative. The Annals of Thoracic Surgery. 1987;**43**(3):326-328

[4] Erdil N, Ates S, Demirkilic U, Tatar H, Sag C. Coronary-coronary bypass using vein graft on a beating heart in a patient with porcelain aorta. Texas Heart Institute Journal. 2002;**29**(1):54-55

[5] Yalcinkaya A, Cagli KE, Ulas MM, Okten SR, Cagli K. Coronary-coronary bypass grafting to reduce the risk of aortic atheroembolism. Journal of Cardiac Surgery. 2010;**25**(2):167-169

[6] Mariscalco G, Blanzola C, Leva C, Bruno VD, Luvini M, Sala A. 19-year patency of a coronary-coronary venous bypass graft. Texas Heart Institute Journal. 2005;**32**(4):583-585

[7] Tixier DB, Acar C, Carpentier AF. Coronary-coronary bypass using the radial artery. The Annals of Thoracic Surgery. 1995;**60**(3):693-694

[8] Nottin R, Grinda JM, Anidjar S, Folliguet T, Detroux M. Coronary-coronary bypass graft: an arterial conduit-sparing procedure. The Journal of Thoracic and Cardiovascular Surgery. 1996;**12**:1223-1230

[9] Bazylev V, Rosseikin E, Tungusov D, Mikulyak A. Coronary-coronary bypass grafting: artery or vein? Asian Cardiovascular & Thoracic Annals. 2020;**28**(6):316-321

[10] Nakajima M, Tsuchiya K, Okamoto Y, Yano K, Kobayashi T. Coronary-coronary artery bypass for right coronary revascularization in patients undergoing graft replacement of the ascending aorta. Annals of Thoracic and Cardiovascular Surgery. 2009;**15**:58-60

[11] Barboso G, Rusticali F. Proximal internal mammary in situ graft and distal coronary-coronary graft to revascularize left anterior descending coronary artery. Texas Heart Institute Journal. 2000;**27**:70-71

[12] Aazami MH. The difference is meaningful: anatomic coronary-coronary bypass or physiologic coronarycoronary bypass? The Journal of Thoracic and Cardiovascular Surgery. 2004;**128**:799-800

[13] Nezić D, Knezević A, Borović S, Cirković M, Milojević P. Coronary-coronary free internal thoracic artery graft on a single, distal, left anterior descending artery lesion. The Journal of Thoracic and Cardiovascular Surgery. 2004;**127**(5):1517-1518

[14] Bruschke AV, Wijers TS, Kolsters W, Landmann J. The anatomic evolution of coronary artery disease demonstrated by coronary arteriography in 256 nonoperated patients. Circulation. 1981;**63**:527-536

[15] Korkmaz AA, Onan B, Tamtekin B, et al. Right coronary revascularization by coronary–coronary bypass with a segment of internal thoracic artery. Texas Heart Institute Journal. 2007;**34**(170-174):10

Chapter 6

Coronary Arteries Bypass Grafting as a Salvage Surgery in Ischemic Heart Failure

Samuel Jacob, Pankaj Garg, Games Gramm and Saqib Masroor

Abstract

Ischemic cardiomyopathy accounts for approximately two-thirds of all Heart Failure (HF) cases. Recent studies indicates that revascularization provides superior outcomes compared with optimal medical therapy (OMT) alone. Current European and American guidelines recommend an invasive approach in patients with reduced left ventricular ejection fraction (LVEF) less than 35% and with multivessel disease (MVD). Randomized controlled trials in these patients have proven that long-term survival is greater following coronary artery bypass grafting (CABG) than with OMT alone. Patients with ischemic cardiomyopathy and coronary artery disease that is amenable to surgical revascularization should undergo combination of surgical revascularization and medical therapy rather than medical therapy alone. In some cases, combined CABG with other surgeries are vital salvage procedures, such as atrial fibrillation, mitral valve, tricuspid valve, and LV remodeling. Based on small but, nontrivial, early mortality risk associated with CABG surgery as well as other post-CABG morbidities, patients may also reasonably choose medical therapy as initial treatment option. Revascularization remains an important treatment option for patients with ongoing anginal symptoms despite optimal medical therapy. In this chapter, we will highlight the role of CABG in heart failure treatment and when to use it as a salvage surgery before referring the patient for heart transplantation.

Keywords: CABG, ischemic heart failure, cardiac surgery, salvage surgery, cardiomyopathy, combined CABG and MVR, combined CABG and TVR, ventricular remodeling

1. Introduction

There is no universally accepted definition of ischemic cardiomyopathy (ICM). However, the term ischemic cardiomyopathy generally refers to significantly impaired left ventricular function (left ventricular ejection fraction [LVEF] ≤35–40%) that results from coronary artery disease (CAD) [1–3]. In 2002, Felker et al. suggested that the symptomatic patients with LVEF ≤40% and presence of left main or proximal left anterior descending coronary artery stenosis ≥75% or two or more epicardial coronary artery stenosis ≥75% or a prior history of coronary artery revascularization [percutaneous coronary intervention (PCI) or coronary artery

IntechOpen

bypass grafting (CABG)] or prior history of myocardial infarction should only be classified as having ICM [3].

Ischemic heart disease is a global pandemic, and its incidence continues to increase. In an estimate, 125 million people across the globe suffer from ischemic heart disease. In the United States itself, every year 720,000 people develop their first myocardial infarction (MI) resulting in hospitalization and/or death [4, 5]. Thirty-five percent of the patients who experience coronary event in a given year die due to it; and each death is associated with an average of 16 years of lost life. Patients who survive after the myocardial infarction are at an increased risk of developing ICM and eventually heart failure (HF). Etiopathogenesis of heart failure is multifactorial; however, ischemic cardiomyopathy is the single most common cause of heart failure. More than 64.3 million people across the world and 6 million people in the United States currently experience HF [3, 6]. In addition to increase in human toll, the estimated cost of HF exceeds $60 billion each year [7, 8].

2. Pathophysiology of ischemic cardiomyopathy

In patients with coronary artery disease, rupture of atherosclerotic plaque followed by in situ thrombus formation leads to sudden cessation of coronary blood flow. If the coronary blood flow is not established early enough either by spontaneous, pharmacological, or interventional recanalization, the death of ischemic myocytes ensues. With time, dead myocytes are replaced with fibrous tissue. Once the amount of scarred myocardium is significant enough after single or multiple episodes of MI, the left ventricle remodels with dilatation, regional deformation, and decrease in overall contractility. Remodeling and alteration of LV geometry especially the inferior wall may also lead to papillary muscle malalignment and mitral regurgitation (MR). Left ventricle volume overloading due to chronic MR in association with poor left ventricular contractility sets up a vicious cycle of worsening LV remodeling and MR [9].

The replacement of the dead myocardium with fibrous tissue is the most important mechanism in the development of ICM. Other pathophysiological processes such as myocardial stunning and hibernation that render the viable myocardial cells unable to perform their mechanical work and also contribute to the development of ICM. Both myocardial stunning and hibernation are reversible forms of myocardial contractile dysfunction that have the potential of mechanical work restoration if the blood flow supply can be improved [10]. In any given heart with ICM, all three stages of myocardium, i.e., normal, viable but hypocontractile and scarred myocardium often coexist within a single cross section of LV. Thus, ischemic cardiomyopathy is extremely heterogeneous and particularly challenging for accurate viability assessment with imaging studies [11].

The concept of hibernating myocardium is interesting as well as mysterious. Our present understanding about the hibernating myocardium is limited [12–16]. Rahimtoola [17] described the hibernating myocardium as "resting left ventricular dysfunction due to reduced coronary blood flow that can be partially or completely reversed by myocardial revascularization and/or by reducing myocardial oxygen demand." Hibernating myocardium is usually limited to subendocardial tissues. Histologically, in hibernating myocardium, there is loss of contractile proteins and sarcoplasmic reticulum without the change in the cell volume. Presumably, hibernation is a protective dedifferentiation of myocardial cells or switch to a quiescent state of decreased mechanical work in times of chronically decreased oxygen supply [13]. This adaptive mechanism probably allows the myocytes to avoid the ischemic imbalance and remain alive in the milieu of decreased coronary blood flow that would otherwise lead to cell death. Alternative mechanism for ventricular dysfunction in ICM may be myocardial stunning. Myocardial stunning apparently occurs due to repeated episodes of ischemic insult that result in viable but chronically hypocontractile myocardium (i.e., repetitive stunning). Due to extremely low ischemic threshold of the myocytes, any decrease in coronary blood flow during stress leads to ischemia and ischemia–reperfusion changes in the myocytes despite normal or insignificantly decreased resting coronary perfusion [13, 18]. This repetitive stunning of the myocytes results in chronic LV dysfunction. Thus, in patients with ICM, territories with high numbers of cardiomyocytes with excess glycogen reserve and less fibrosis in all probabilities are reversible after revascularization. These myocytes also demonstrate higher blood flow and glucose uptake on positron emission tomography (PET) scan [19].

3. Preoperative considerations

Patients with ICM present with myriad of signs and symptoms depending upon the severity of heart failure and degree of physiological compensation. Some patients may be asymptomatic or minimally symptomatic with mild anginal chest pain and dyspnea on exertion while other patients may present with overt heart failure symptoms, e.g., dyspnea, orthopnea, poor exercise tolerance, and increased fatigability. Patients usually have a longstanding history of coronary artery disease and a prior history of myocardial infarctions. Physical examination can reveal bibasilar crackles, S3 gallop, displaced apical impulse, carotid bruits, jugular venous distension, positive hepato-jugular reflex, and bilateral lower extremity edema.

3.1 Diagnostic testing

In patients with ICM, multivessel disease, low LVEF, and increased LV end-systolic volumes are important prognostic factors. Therefore, all these factors must be taken into consideration when making the difficult decision regarding revascularization. Suitability of the patient for CABG depends upon: A) suitability of the diseased coronary arteries for bypass grafting; B) the amount of viable myocardium present and whether the viable myocardium is present in the territory of CAD; C) severity of right and left heart failure; and D) associated cardiac lesions. All the diagnostic investigations should be directed toward determining whether the patient is a suitable candidate for CABG or not.

Transthoracic echocardiography (TTE): Transthoracic echocardiography is an essential investigation in assessing myocardial viability in a patient with ICM. Echocardiography is useful in evaluating cardiac anatomy, valvular function, ventricular systolic/diastolic function, cardiac wall motion, and pericardial pathology. All this information is useful in diagnosing ischemic cardiomyopathy, especially in patients with HF and other high-risk features.

Coronary angiography: Coronary angiography allows direct visualization of the coronary arteries for assessment of severity of obstruction, collateralization, and the blood flow to the myocardium. Coronary angiography is most important in defining the extent and severity of coronary artery disease and whether the coronaries arteries are suitable for grafting. Computed tomography coronary angiography can also be performed in place of conventional coronary angiography to assess coronary arteries in patients with low to intermediate risk of CAD [20].

Cardiac stress test: There are different stress tests available depending on the patient's health, functional status, baseline heart rhythm, and exercise tolerance. The goal of these stress tests is to assess for cardiac ischemia and myocardial viability. Late gadolinium enhancement cardiac magnetic resonance (LGE-CMR), dobutamine stress echocardiography, single-photon emission computed tomography (SPECT), and F-18- fluorodeoxyglucose positron emission tomography (FDG-PET) imaging can be used to assess myocardial viability [21]. Dobutamine stress echocardiography is widely used to assess myocardial contractility reserve and viability. With continuous dobutamine infusion, initially myocardial perfusion increases along with increased contractility. However, as the dobutamine dose increases, blood flow cannot be escalated further leading to reduced myocardial contractility. This phenomenon known as biphasic reaction can predict the recovery of the myocardial function after revascularization.

Late gadolinium enhancement cardiovascular magnetic resonance (LGE-CMR) can detect increase in extracellular space due to myocardial apoptosis and necrosis and can predict the reversibility of the myocardial contractility after successful revascularization while dobutamine stress CMR can detect the ischemic myocardium. In patients with ICM with transmural infarct, minimal LGE (<25%) in dysfunctional myocardial segment indicates a high likelihood of recovery while the chance of recovery is minimal in segments with >50% LGE.[13] In segments with 25–50% LGE involvement, the recovery prediction is not consistent [22].

Single-photon emission computed tomography (SPECT) and positron emission tomography (PET) had been widely utilized in the past to assess myocardial viability. Thallium-based SPECT scan demonstrate delayed distribution but has increased risk of ionizing radiations while technetium-based SPECT has less risk of radiation, but it cannot demonstrate a delayed distribution. Another nuclear imaging modality to assess myocardial viability is cardiac PET. PET imaging is based on the principle that in an ICM, ischemic myocardium switches to glucose-based metabolism instead of fatty acids. ^{18}F-fluorodeoxyglucose (^{18}F-FDG) can detect this shift in viable but ischemic myocardium. PET has higher spatial resolution, lower risk of radiation, and better attenuation correction compared with SPECT. PET, however, cannot distinguish between normal and ischemic or hibernating myocardium in patients with insulin resistance, and results may be inaccurate in patients with variable uptake of FDG due to heart failure [23].

Brain natriuretic peptide (BNP) test: BNP is synthesized in the ventricles, and it is secreted when the myocardial muscle has a high wall tension. BNP is an important biomarker for heart failure patients. Increasing trend in BNP suggests worsening of heart failure; however, it cannot detect myocardial ischemia.

4. Clinical studies and randomized trials in patients with ischemic cardiomyopathy

Coronary artery bypass grafting for CAD started in the mid-1960s. Since then, numerous clinical trials and studies have tried to address different questions related to the management of CAD. All these trials and studies have established an undisputed role of surgical revascularization in patients with CAD in terms of improved survival, risk of reintervention, and quality of life [24–27]. Nevertheless, prior to Surgical Treatment for Ischemic Heart Failure (STICH) trial [28], none of the studies specifically addressed the management of patients with ICM. The coronary artery surgery study (CASS) trial registry that followed the patients who were excluded from the main study reported that patients with LVEF <35% had better survival with CABG than with medical therapy, if they had associated three-vessel disease and if the presenting symptom was angina [29]. Similarly, a 25-year observational study involving 1391 patients (medical therapy (n = 1052) or CABG (n = 339)) from Duke Cardiovascular Disease Databank also reported an improved survival with CABG over medical therapy alone after 30 days to more than 10 years in patients with NYHA class ≥II, CAD with at least one vessel stenosis ≥75%, and LVEF <40%. The benefit with CABG was observed irrespective of the extent of coronary artery involvement ($P < 0.001$) [30].

These observational studies pointed toward the role of CABG in patients with ischemic cardiomyopathy; however, lack of randomized clinical studies in patients with ICM led to different therapeutic approaches driven by the physician bias regarding the potential benefit of myocardial revascularization [9]. The resulting equipoise formed the basis for the multiinstitutional STICH randomized controlled clinical trial [28]. STICH trial was the first and only large-scale randomized clinical trial to compare surgical revascularization with medical therapy in patients with LVEF ≤35% and CAD amenable to CABG. The STICH trial randomly assigned 1212 patients to three groups (medical therapy alone, medical therapy with CABG, and medical therapy with CABG and SVR). To evaluate the superiority of either procedure, two hypotheses were developed. In Hypotheses 1, the investigators evaluated medical therapy against medical therapy with CABG. All patients underwent coronary angiography to define the extent of CAD; patients with critical left main disease or unstable coronary syndromes were excluded from the trial. The primary outcome of the study was all-cause mortality, and secondary outcomes were cardiovascular mortality, combination of all-cause mortality and hospitalization for cardiac causes. At a median follow-up of 56 months, medical therapy plus CABG surgery resulted in a nonsignificant trend toward improvement in the primary outcome (36% vs. 41% with medical therapy alone) as well as significantly lower cardiovascular mortality and improved quality of life (at 4, 12, 24, and 36 months as assessed by the Kansas City Cardiomyopathy Questionnaire) [31]. However, this trial was fraught with certain limitations. First, during the study period, 9% patients in medical therapy plus CABG group crossed over to medical therapy group only while 17% patients in medical therapy alone group crossed over to medical therapy and CABG group. This crossover may have led to a diminished treatment benefit, thereby preventing the primary outcome from reaching statistical significance. Second, the STICH trial was designed to maximize both medical and surgical outcomes using strict criteria for surgical expertise (e.g., documented surgical expertise by volume and outcome criteria) and regular review of both surgical center conduct and intensity of medical therapy. Clinical equipoise had to be present, and both the surgeon and cardiologist had to believe revascularization was technically feasible. Both these issues may limit the generalizability of the trial to routine clinical practice.

In 2016, results of extended follow-up of STICH trial patients, i.e., the STICH Extension Study (STICHES), were published extending the median follow-up to 9.8 years [32]. After 9.8 years, the primary outcome (all-cause mortality) was significantly lower in the medical therapy and CABG group compared with medical therapy alone group (59% vs. 66%; hazard ratio [HR] 0.84; 95% CI, 0.73–0.97). Medical therapy and CABG group also experienced significant reductions in cardiovascular mortality (40.5% vs. 49.3%; HR 0.79; 95% CI, 0.66–0.93) and the combination of all-cause mortality and cardiovascular hospitalization (76.6% vs. 87%; HR 0.72; 95% CI, 0.64–0.82). Another large population based observational study related to CAD with LV systolic dysfunction was reported [33], it is recommended to do CABG and medical therapy for patients with ICM who have coronaries amenable to surgical revascularization.

5. Myocardial viability and treatment decisions

Observational studies done in early 2000s focused on the potential benefit of viable myocardium on the patient survival and LV function after the revascularization. Initial potential survival benefit from revascularization in patients with ICM and viable myocardium was reported in a meta-analysis published in 2002. This meta-analysis included 24 nonrandomized viability studies involving 3088 patients with CAD and LV dysfunction who had a mean LVEF of 32% [34]. Patients with myocardial viability had 80% reduction in annual mortality with revascularization (3.2% vs. 16% with medical therapy alone), while there was no significant change in annual mortality with revascularization in patients without myocardial viability (7.7% vs. 6.2% with medical therapy alone). Potential effect of viable myocardium on LVEF was also illustrated in a review published in 2004 that involved 29 observational studies including 758 patients [35]. In this review, LVEF increased after revascularization when myocardial viability was present (37–45%) but did not change significantly in the absence of viability. Further, studies have also demonstrated that 25–30% of the dysfunctional myocardium needs to be viable to result in improvement of LVEF. On the contrary, in a substudy of the STICH trial, 601 of the 1212 patients were evaluated for myocardial viability, and outcomes were analyzed according to those assigned to receive medical therapy plus CABG or medical therapy alone. Study showed minimal improvement in LVEF with revascularization (from 28% pre-CABG to 30% post-CABG). Following adjustment for differences in baseline variables and with follow-up extending beyond 10 years, there was no significant improvement in mortality with medical therapy plus CABG compared with medical therapy alone. Myocardial viability was associated with reduced mortality but did not predict a benefit from revascularization. This raises the question of whether viability assessment is needed prior to surgical revascularization. However, myocardial viability in STICH trial was assessed using stress echocardiography and SPECT radionuclide myocardial perfusion imaging; more contemporary techniques such as CMR and positron emission tomography (PET) were not studied and are an important limitation of the STICH findings [36]. Presence of myocardial viability does lead to improvement in contractility and myocardial thickness following revascularization subject to the presence of at least 25–30% of viable myocardium and scar burden <25% (as detected by LGE-CMR) [37]. However, inconsistencies in the criteria and the methods used to diagnose myocardial viability between various studies have led to blurring of the evidence of benefit of revascularization.

In the absence of firm evidence, routine viability assessment prior to consideration for CABG in patients with ICM is not recommended. However, situations that require greater precision in defining large infarcts either due to associated excessive surgical morbidity (e.g., renal failure) or risk of suboptimal outcome (e.g., evidence of LV remodeling, inability to achieve complete revascularization); viability assessment with more contemporary techniques such as LGE-CMR or FDG-PET may help further refine the potential risks and benefits.

6. Impact of left ventricular size and remodeling

Left ventricular size is an important determinant of outcome after surgical revascularization in patients with ICM. However, our present understanding of impact of preoperative LV size on postoperative LV function and survival is still limited. The impact of left ventricular enlargement on the improvement in LV function after revascularization was illustrated in a review of 61 patients with ischemic heart disease and a mean LVEF of 28%, all of whom had an evidence of substantial myocardial viability [38]. One-third of the patients had no significant improvement in the LVEF (≥5%). The study showed that the patients with a significant improvement in LVEF after CABG had a significantly smaller left ventricular end-systolic volume (LVESV) on preoperative echocardiography than those without improvement (121 mL vs. 153 mL). The observational data are in contrast with the findings from the STICH trial, which found greater benefit with respect to mortality in patients with greater baseline remodeling (e.g., larger left ventricle end-systolic volume index [LVESVI]) [28].

7. Percutaneous coronary intervention versus surgical revascularization

Percutaneous coronary intervention (PCI) is an established treatment for revascularization in acute myocardial infarction. Role of PCI in management of ICM is still unclear due to the lack of well-designed randomized studies. In the lack of randomized controlled study, best available data come from the observational study comparing PCI with CABG in 4616 patients with LVEF ≤35% who were enrolled in New York State registries (1351 underwent PCI with drug eluting stents and 3265 underwent CABG), from which 2126 patients were chosen for evaluation based on propensity score matching [39]. At a median follow-up of 2.9 years, there was no significant difference in mortality between contemporary PCI and CABG (HR 1.01; 95% CI 0.81–1.28). PCI was associated with a greater risk of myocardial infarction (HR 2.16; 95% CI 1.42–3.28) and need for repeat revascularization (HR 2.54; 95% CI 1.88–3.44), but a significantly lower risk of stroke compared with CABG (HR 0.57; 95% CI 0.33–0.97).

In a separate post hoc analysis of AWESOME trial, in which 454 patients who had medically refractory unstable or provocable ischemia were randomized to PCI or CABG. Ninety-four patients had LVEF <35% (mean 25%) [40]. Among patients with LVEF <35%, there was no difference in mortality between CABG and PCI. However, limitation of this trial was that all patients included in the study had angina and acute coronary syndromes and not heart failure.

8. Role of CABG in patients with ischemic cardiomyopathy

The mechanism of survival advantage conferred by CABG in patients with heart failure irrespective of myocardial viability still remains speculative, although, post hoc analysis of STICH trial has been able to shed some interesting insight on this topic. In STICH trial, a subanalysis evaluating cause-specific cardiac mortality in patients with ICM demonstrated that sudden cardiac death (SCD) was the most frequent mode of death and outnumbered pump failure deaths by approximately two-fold [41]. Further, both SCD and death from HF were significantly reduced after the CABG (as was death from myocardial infarction). Predictors of increased risk of SCD in this analysis were increased LVESVI and elevated BNP level. Interestingly, same variables along with regional myocardial sympathetic denervation were found to be significant risk factors for SCD in patients with ICM in the Prediction of Arrhythmic Events with Positron Emission Tomography (PAREPET) Study [42, 43]. Thus, the survival benefit of CABG in patients with ICM is largely due to the significant effect of revascularization on reducing the death due to arrhythmia with a smaller contribution from reducing the deaths from pump failure and fatal MI.

9. Our approach to patients with ischemic cardiomyopathy

We suggest the combined CABG and medical therapy instead of medical therapy alone for patients with ICM and CAD that is amenable to surgical revascularization. This suggestion is based primarily on a 7% absolute reduction in overall mortality over 10 years (STICH trial) and superior relief of anginal symptoms following CABG. However, as significant morbidity and early mortality (compared with medical management alone) are associated with CABG in patients with ICM, patients may also reasonably choose medical therapy alone as the initial treatment option. Following initiation of medical therapy, patients should be reevaluated on an ongoing basis for any changes in clinical status or symptoms and consideration for surgical revascularization should be discussed with the patient.

Other clinical features that should be considered while tailoring the decision for any given patient are greater functional capacity (6-minute walk >300 m), greater burden of CAD (e.g., three-vessel disease), coexistent moderate to severe mitral regurgitation (MR), lower ejection fraction (e.g., LVEF <35%), and greater remodeling (e.g., LVESVI >79 mL/m^2) (associated with improved outcomes in STICH trial).

Additionally, we do not recommend routine viability assessment prior to consideration for surgical revascularization and consideration should be case-to-case basis especially in patients in whom the risk-to-benefit profile is not as clear (e.g., patients with significantly elevated surgical risk). We believe that viability study may not aid in decision-making; however, the presence of significant viability and < 25–30% scar on LGE-CMR gives reassurance to the surgeon for improved surgical outcome.

Considering the advantage with CABG from the STICHES trial, it seems that patients with suitable targets for revascularization in the setting of an EF < 35% with two or three vessel CAD should be considered for CABG irrespective of the results of viability testing. However, competing risk factors such as severity of heart failure, age of the patient, and risks for noncardiac mortality need to be carefully weighed in considering the recommendation for revascularization and decision should be made on individual basis.

10. Preoperative optimization and perioperative temporary mechanical support

Factors that have been consistently associated with adverse outcomes after CABG for patients with ICM include preoperative renal dysfunction, advanced HF, recent myocardial infarction, and hemodynamic instability. Perioperative shock in this patient population more than doubles the rate of perioperative mortality [44–46]. Therefore, preoperative optimization of the patient status can improve the patient outcome after the surgery. The specific mode of optimization should be individualized to patients' needs and driven by their response to initial therapy. If medical therapy alone is ineffective, more invasive measures should be considered. In the preoperative setting, prophylactic intra-aortic balloon pump (IABP) decreases afterload, increases coronary artery perfusion, provides a modest increase in cardiac output [47, 48]. In a variety of analyses, IABP therapy before the operation has been noted to result not only in improved patient condition before CABG, but also in reduced perioperative morbidity and mortality. Two meta-analyses of randomized clinical trials examining the utility of preoperative IABP therapy in patients with ICM demonstrated a strong association between preoperative use of IABP and reduced hospital mortality, lower incidence of low cardiac output syndrome, and shorter duration of ICU stay. Patients with high-risk profile including low LVEF, left main disease >70%, prior heart surgery, poor coronary artery targets, and unstable angina typically benefit from preoperative IABP [47–50].

In patients who present with cardiogenic shock resulting from acute myocardial infarction or decompensated HF with end-organ dysfunction, IABP may be inadequate for stabilization or preoperative optimization. In these patients, transvalvular devices such as microaxial surgical heart pump can be used. These devices reduce left ventricular end-diastolic pressure (LVEDP) and volume workload and provide the circulatory support necessary to allow native heart recovery. In a recent analysis, the use of these micro-axial pump was associated with reduced mortality, without significant increase in device-related stroke, hemolysis, or limb ischemia [51, 52]. Finally, in patients with cardiogenic shock that is refractory to inotropic support, IABP, and/or microaxial pumps, ventricular assist device (VAD) implantation should be considered [47, 53, 54].

Patients with ICM with cardiogenic shock, who have organ dysfunction at the time of presentation, temporary VAD can be used as bridge to decision. Patients who reverse their organ dysfunction and acidosis after the insertion of temporary MCS and demonstrate an adequate contractile reserve and response to inotropic stimulation can successfully bridge to CABG. This is contingent to good coronary targets and absence of unfavorable anatomic and physiologic profiles [27]. Otherwise, they should be evaluated for heart transplant and should be considered for more durable VAD option as bridge to transplant.

11. Coronary artery bypass graft surgery strategy

11.1 On-pump arrested-heart CABG

The goal of CABG in patients with ICM is to achieve expeditious and complete revascularization. On-pump arrested-heart CABG is the most commonly used strategy that allows a bloodless and still field that facilitates complete revascularization [55]. Excellent myocardial protection especially right ventricle is paramount in the setting of ischemic cardiomyopathy as myocardial ischemia and injury are poorly tolerated when myocardial reserve is limited [56].

In patients undergoing on-pump CABG, controversy still remains about type of cardioplegic solution, temperature, and route of administration that provides the optimal myocardial protection. This becomes critical in patients with ICM as any amount of further myocardial damage may be deleterious. In a meta-analysis of 12 studies including 2866 patients, lower prevalence of perioperative myocardial infarction was found in patients who received blood cardioplegia [57]. Another meta-analysis of 41 randomized clinical trials (RCT) found that warm cardioplegia did not improve clinical outcomes but was associated with a mild reduction of cardiac enzyme release [58]. Single-dose cardioplegia benefit is limited to a reduction in ischemia and bypass time and does not translate into a major morbidity or mortality advantage [59]. There is no systematic comparison of different routes of cardioplegia administration (i.e., antegrade vs. retrograde vs. combined); however, isolated retrograde cardioplegia should be avoided due to its heterogeneous perfusion and unpredictable right ventricle myocardial protection [60]. On the other hand, retrograde cardioplegia may be useful in adjunct to antegrade cardioplegia in patients with severe CAD and in redo CABG to reach territories not otherwise reachable by antegrade delivery and to flush potential embolic debris from inadvertently manipulated diseased vein grafts [61, 62]. Although data are scarce, it has been reported that antegrade cardioplegia supplemented with venous graft perfusion can significantly improve myocardial protection. The most suitable myocardial protection strategy may be a combination of antegrade, retrograde, and delivery down the vein grafts.

11.2 Off-pump CABG

Utilization of off-pump CABG (OPCABG) is limited to few centers and selected patients in the developed countries. There have been no large RCTs comparing on-pump CABG versus OPCABG and small RCTs that did compare these two modalities have reported inferior or non-superior long-term outcome with OPCABG. Most of these studies are limited by smaller sample size, short duration of follow-up, and limited experience of the operator. This is of particular relevance given that OPCABG may lead to inferior long-term outcomes if performed by inexperienced operators and/or accompanied by incomplete revascularization [63]. In a meta-analysis of 23 individual nonrandomized studies published in 2011 that involved 7759 CABG patients with LVEF <40%, 2822 patients underwent OPCABG. Overall early mortality was significantly reduced (odds ratio [OR], 0.64; 95% CI, 0.51–0.81) in OPCABG group. Similar results were observed on subgroup analysis of 1915 patients with LVEF <30% (OR 0.61; 95% CI 0.47–0.80) [64]. A recent meta-analysis published in 2020 comprising 16 studies with 32,354 patients with LV dysfunction (defined as LVEF <40%) also reported a significant reduction in 30-day mortality (OR 0.84; 95% CI 0.73–0.97), perioperative complications, and transfusion requirements with OPCABG [65]. In a report published in 2016 from the Japan Adult Cardiovascular Surgery Database including 918 pairs of propensity-matched CABG patients with LVEF <30%, there was reduced perioperative and 30-day mortality with OPCABG (1.7% vs. 3.7%; $P < 0.01$) and reduced incidence of mediastinitis, reoperation for bleeding, and need for prolonged ventilation, but there was no difference in incidence of stroke or renal failure compared to on-pump CABG [66].

11.3 On-pump beating-heart CABG

On-pump beating-heart CABG has been proposed as an alternative strategy to on-pump cardioplegic arrest CABG, particularly in higher-risk patients including patients with impaired LV function [67]. This technique is more of historical significance as it is rarely used nowadays. In a review of 11 studies, comprising two RCTs and nine observational studies comparing on-pump beating-heart CABG and on-pump arrested heart CABG, lower mortality was reported with on-pump beating-heart CABG in five of the nine observational studies while mortality was similar with both techniques in two RCTs. However, due to the lack of randomization and the absence of propensity matching, the possibility of selection bias accounting for the difference in mortality cannot be discounted. Intraoperative myocardial injury with on-pump beating heart may increase due to inadequate coronary perfusion distal to areas of stenosis [68].

In the absence of more definitive evidence about the superiority of one technique of CABG over the other, the operative strategy should be tailored based on patient factors such as extent of CAD and associated comorbidities, surgeon's expertise and comfort level of the cardiac anesthetist, and center experience. When off-pump technique is used, maintenance of appropriate perfusion pressure and when on-pump CABG is utilized, appropriate myocardial protection is imperative to minimize further myocardial injury.

12. Bypass conduits

Presently, use of left internal mammary artery (LIMA) for bypassing left anterior descending coronary artery and reverse saphenous vein grafts for bypassing rest of the coronary arteries is the standard of care across the globe. Evidence from the recent studies has shown the superiority of multi-arterial grafting in improving long-term patient survival after CABG. The impact on survival becomes even more significant with increasing duration of follow-up [69–71]. The evidence of beneficial effects of multi-arterial grafting in patients with ICM, however, is limited to few studies and a small number of patients [72–74]. Further, multi-arterial grafting in patients with ICM still remains controversial as the overriding priority in these patients is to mitigate the upfront risk of surgery and avoidance of perioperative myocardial ischemia. In a risk predictive model based on STS database review of patients operated for CABG, the HR for perioperative mortality after isolated CABG was 1.19 (95% CI, 1.17–1.22) for every 10% reduction in LVEF [75], and operative risk was further compounded with the addition of noncardiac organ dysfunction and other comorbidities.

There are four reasons why caution should be used when contemplating multi-arterial grafting in patients with ICM [56]. First, perioperative administration of high doses of vasopressors may be necessary in these patients, and this is an important predisposing factor for the development of spasm in the arterial grafts [76]. Radial and gastroepiploic arteries are particularly vulnerable to spasm compared with IMAs. Second, adequacy of blood flow in a fresh arterial graft may not be as robust as in a vein graft, with the potential for clinically significant perioperative coronary artery hypoperfusion [77–79]. Third, multi-arterial grafting usually adds to the complexity and length of the operation and prolongs myocardial ischemic time. This may not be well tolerated by the patients with ICM. Fourth, arterial grafts may not be of adequate length in massively dilated hearts, especially if sequential anastomoses are contemplated. A patient-level combined analysis of six RCTs associated radial artery grafts in addition to LIMA with improved clinical outcomes compared with venous grafts [80]. The benefit of radial artery grafting was persistent even on subgroup analysis of patients with severe LV dysfunction (LVEF <35%). However, the number of patients in subgroup were limited (25 (4.7%) and 32 (6.4%) in the radial artery and saphenous vein groups, respectively). The results of other observational studies have yielded mixed results with the use of multi-arterial grafting in patients with ICM [73, 81–84]. The probable reason is variable cutoff for LVEF with different studies (lowest limit <30%), which adds to uncertainty regarding multi-arterial grafting benefits [85]. Observational evidence also suggests that the benefit of multi-arterial grafting is lost in patients with ICM with limited life expectancy or severe associated comorbidities [83, 86–88].

We believe that multi-arterial grafting should not be routinely recommended for patients with ICM. Patient selection for multi-arterial grafting should be based on patient factors and surgeon's experience and comfort. Young patients with compensated HF having good target for bypass may be considered for multi-arterial grafting if the risk–benefit ratio is favorable and prolonged survival is anticipated after revascularization.

13. CABG combined with other procedures

13.1 Atrial fibrillation

Atrial fibrillation (AFib) is present in 5–10% of patients undergoing CABG. It is associated with increased risk of complications including stroke and renal failure, prolonged hospital stay as well as increased mortality despite adjustment for potential confounders [89]. Therefore, current North American and European guidelines for CABG recommend concomitant AFib ablation procedure in symptomatic patients or asymptomatic patients having low operative risk [90, 91]. The evidence supporting the surgical ablation of AFib in patients with ICM undergoing CABG is minimal and limited by selection bias [92]. Theoretically, patients with a reduced ejection fraction would benefit from the restoration of sinus rhythm and atrial contraction [93]. However, concomitant AFib ablation procedure adds to the technical complexity of the surgery and prolongs the duration of aortic cross clamp and cardiopulmonary bypass. Despite this, some studies reported that surgical AFib ablation is safe and effective in patients with heart failure [94, 95].

13.2 Mitral valve surgery

Up to 10% patients develop chronic moderate or severe MR following acute myocardial infarction. Chronic ischemic mitral regurgitation (CIMR) is associated with an increased incidence of heart failure and increased risk of mortality in patients with LV dysfunction [96]. Furthermore, LV dysfunction can lead to gradual dilatation and geometric change in the left ventricle that results in distortion of the mitral valve and worsening of MR. Although, there is a general consensus to repair or replace the mitral valve in patients with severe CIMR undergoing CABG, the management of moderate (Grade II) mitral regurgitation still remains controversial.

In the Cardiothoracic Surgical Trials Network study, adding surgical mitral valve repair to CABG in patients with moderate CIMR had no significant effect on survival or LV reverse remodeling at 2 years follow-up but was associated with increased duration of hospital stay and morbidity including neurological events and atrial arrhythmias [97]. Smaller RCTs have shown benefit in surrogate outcomes for CABG and mitral valve repair versus CABG alone in patients with moderate CIMR [98, 99]. However, none of the trials has specifically focused on patients with ICM. In patients with severe CIMR, mitral valve replacement has been shown to provide more reliable and durable relief of MR than repair, but without survival benefit [100]. Mitral valve replacement rather than repair is also favored in patients with LV basal aneurysm/dyskinesis or other potential risk factors for recurrent MR after repair, e.g., significant leaflet tethering and/or severe left ventricular dilatation (LV end-diastolic dimension >6.5 cm). Preserving the subvalvular apparatus is also strongly recommended when replacing mitral valve in these patients. Concerns about persistent tethering of the posterior leaflet and recurrent MR after CABG in patients with prior inferior wall MI have prompted some to combine mitral anuloplasty with a subvalvular procedure such as papillary muscle approximation and papillary muscle relocation. All these procedures result in improved echocardiographic and cardiovascular outcomes but fail to influence all-cause mortality or quality of life [101–103]. Therefore, this remains an area for further study and evaluation.

13.3 Tricuspid valve surgery

Tricuspid regurgitation (TR) is an established risk factor in patients undergoing CABG [104]. In patients with CIMR, although progression of unrepaired mild to moderate TR after revascularization is uncommon, presence and progression of moderate or greater TR are associated with increased incidence of clinical events [105]. The underlying etiology of TR in ICM includes tricuspid annular dilatation and leaflet tethering in the setting of RV remodeling due to right ventricle infarction with or without pulmonary hypertension, tricuspid annular dilatation associated with AFib, and iatrogenic or lead related injury to tricuspid leaflets. Current AHA/ACC guidelines assign class I recommendation for tricuspid valve repair at the time of left sided valve surgery for severe TR and class IIa for less than severe TR in the presence of annular dilatation (>4.0 cm) or right-sided HF [106].

Concomitant mitral valve repair can be considered in patients with ICM undergoing CABG in the presence of atrial arrhythmias, left atrial dilation, or in the setting of severe LV dilation. Replacement, rather than repair, should be considered in patients with limited viability in the posterolateral wall of the LV [97]. Tricuspid valve repair should be considered at the time of left sided valve surgery for severe TR and less than severe TR in the presence of annular dilatation (>4.0 cm), right-sided HF or iatrogenic, or lead-related injury to tricuspid leaflets. Severe TR in the presence of significant RV dysfunction is a marker of poor outcome after coronary revascularization and warrants evaluation and consideration for advanced HF therapies.

13.4 Surgical ventricular restoration

In patients with ICM, gradual dilatation of LV results in transition from elliptical to a more spherical geometry. This impairs the structure–function relationship of the left ventricle [107]. The concept of surgical ventricular restoration (SVR) procedure for the patients with ICM is more than four decades old; however, the procedure is yet to gain acceptance as not only the procedure is technically challenging but also, no study so far has been able to show consistent benefit with concomitant SVR. Doctrine of SVR operation assumes that resection of scarred myocardium, reducing the ventricular size, and restoring an anatomically elliptical shape can improve the left ventricular function [108]. However, studies so far have not been able to prove this assumption. A randomized study including 137 patients with LVEF <50% and LV end systolic volume index (LVESVI) >80 ml/m^2 showed that CABG alone was inferior to

CABG with SVR in terms of improvement in LVEF, MR, and NYHA class. However, study was limited to only 2 years of follow-up [109]. Similarly, Prucz et al. reported this result [110]. Both these studies were limited by short duration of follow-up and failed to show any benefit of SVR procedure on survival. Consequently, the STICH trial was conducted to evaluate the long-term outcome of concomitant SVR procedure in patients with LV dysfunction, LV akinesis/dyskinesis, presence of scar, and LV dilatation [111]. To evaluate the benefit of SVR, patients enrolled in STICH trial in CABG arm were divided into two groups (medical therapy with CABG versus medical therapy with CABG and SVR). The study found no difference in mortality between the groups at median follow-up of 48 months (hazard ratio 1.00, 95% CI 0.79–1.26, P = 0.98) [111]. Results of these studies led to abandonment of the SVR procedure by majority surgeons [112].

It still remains uncertain which patients should receive SVR as part of CABG operation and what is its impact on long-term survival and functional outcome [112–114]. Therefore, consideration for SVR should still be given to patients with true large ventricular aneurysms who present with medically refractory heart failure or ventricular arrhythmias.

14. Postcardiotomy shock and temporary MCS

Patients with ICM undergoing CABG are at increased risk of postcardiotomy shock and the risk increases further in patients with ischemic MR and/or right ventricular infarct. Patients with postcardiotomy shock who are unable to separate from cardiopulmonary bypass or require high-dose inotropic therapy, MCS should be considered [115].

14.1 Intra-aortic balloon pump (IABP)

Intra-aortic balloon pump has been considered as first line therapy for PCS as it is safe, widely available, and easy to place. Intra-aortic balloon pump improves the coronary perfusion, decreases the left ventricular afterload, and improves the cardiac output by 0.5–1 L/min. However, the hemodynamic support provided by an IABP is usually insufficient in reversing cardiogenic shock [116, 117]. In a recent analysis of 4550 patients operated for CABG between 2004 and 2008, 5% patients required an intraoperative or postoperative IABP, with overall mortality of 37%. IABP was equally effective in patients with predominantly right-sided failure with 50% increase in cardiac index and associated mortality of 31%. This study specifically addressed the issue of IABP effectiveness in both right- and left-sided failure [118].

14.2 Impella

Impella is a percutaneous or surgically implanted axial-flow device that is used for all types of cardiogenic shock. Impella devices significantly reduce LV end-diastolic pressure and volume, reduce myocardial oxygen demand, and support the systemic perfusion while allowing the heart to recover. Engstrom and colleagues [119] reported their experience with Impella 5.0 for treating 46 postcardiotomy shock patients mostly after CABG at three European centers. Half of the patients received an IABP before the Impella placement. Overall survival was 40% at 30 days. More recently, David and colleagues [120] reported on use of the Impella 5.0/Impella LD in 29 patients (40% with isolated CABG) treated for PCS between 2010 and 2015. Mortality was nearly 40%, similar to the aforementioned study. The best results for PCS treatment were reported by Griffith and colleagues [121] in the RECOVER I study, wherein an Impella 5.0 was placed in 16 patients having difficulty weaning from cardiopulmonary bypass. Fifteen patients were successfully supported, with 30-day survival of 94%. Results of this study should however be interpreted carefully as all the patients in the study were on low level of inotropic support before the Impella placement as opposed to the study protocol requirement of high inotropic support prior to Impella placement.

14.3 Extracorporeal membrane oxygenation

Veno-arterial extracorporeal membrane oxygenation (VA-ECMO) is second most commonly used device after IABP for postcardiotomy shock. Veno-arterial ECMO significantly unloads the right ventricle, improves the coronary perfusion, and supports the systemic perfusion while allowing the right heart to recover. However, VA-ECMO significantly increases the left ventricular afterload. Therefore, in patients supported with VA-ECMO, it is imperative to maintain left ventricular ejection either spontaneous or with inotropes. Otherwise, left side of the heart should be vented either by atrial septostomy, left atrial/left ventricular vent, or Impella [122]. There are no RCTs regarding the effectiveness of VA-ECMO in PCS, but several retrospective studies have shown 60–70% mortality in patients with PCS despite use of VA-ECMO [122–125]. In a recent report of the European registry of 781 patients receiving VA-ECMO for PCS, institution of VA-ECMO was associated with increased mortality (odds ratio 1.54; 95% CI, 1.09–2.18), reoperation for bleeding/tamponade (odds ratio, 1.96; 95% CI, 1.37–2.81), and blood transfusion of >9 units (odds ratio, 2.42; 95% CI, 1.59–3.67). The authors also did a systematic review of 2491 patients with PCS who received VA-ECMO and reported 66.6% pooled prevalence of in-hospital/30-day mortality (95% CI, 64.7–68.4%), and lower in-hospital/30-day mortality in patients with peripheral ECMO (risk ratio, 0.92; 95% CI, 0.87–0.98). Switching the patients from central to peripheral cannulation appeared to provide close to a 10% mortality benefit [126]. Finally, studies evaluating the role of LV unloading during VA-ECMO for cardiogenic shock have reported 10–20% mortality benefit with LV unloading with either Impella or IABP [127, 128].

15. Post discharge management

In patients with ICM, the importance of adhering to guideline-directed medical therapy (GDMT), secondary prevention, and cardiac rehabilitation after revascularization cannot be overemphasized [129, 130]. Close follow-up of these patients is recommended for the titration of heart failure medications and continued assessment for needed additional interventions, including device implantation (e.g., automated implantable cardioverter-defibrillator (AICD)/Cardiac resynchronization therapy device (CRT) or advanced surgical therapies for persistent HF. In patients with ICM, initial 90 days after CABG are most vulnerable and associated with several-fold increase in HF-associated rehospitalization and mortality. Thus, these patients should undergo a close clinical monitoring after discharge. Initial post-discharge follow-up should be done at 7–14 days to review the volume status of the patient and titrate guideline-directed medications [131]. Although studies directly evaluating and comparing the impact of GDMT on ICM patients who have or have not undergone CABG are limited, conventional medical opinion supports that GDMT goals for post-CABG patients should not differ from those without CABG. Post hoc analysis has revealed that in patients with ICM, maintenance of optimal medical therapy after discharge is associated with best short-term and long-term outcomes [132].

16. Summary

Patients with ischemic cardiomyopathy and coronary artery disease that is amenable to surgical revascularization should undergo combination of surgical revascularization and medical therapy rather than medical therapy alone. This suggestion is based primarily on the long-term absolute reduction in mortality over the 10 years following CABG balanced against the early mortality risk of CABG. Routine assessment of viability to evaluate advisability of multivessel coronary revascularization to improve total mortality is not recommended. Based on the small but nontrivial early mortality risk associated with CABG surgery as well as other post-CABG morbidities, patients may also reasonably choose medical therapy as the initial treatment option. Revascularization remains an important treatment option for patients with ongoing anginal symptoms despite optimal medical therapy. For such patients, the relative efficacy of percutaneous coronary intervention (PCI) compared with CABG for revascularization is unknown. Nonrandomized registry suggests that there was no difference in mortality between CABG and PCI.

Author details

Samuel Jacob[1]*, Pankaj Garg[2], Games Gramm[3] and Saqib Masroor[4]

1 Clinical Research Director of Cardiothoracic Surgery, Mayo Clinic, Florida, USA

2 Cardiothoracic Surgery, Mayo Clinic, Florida, USA

3 Cardiothoracic Surgery, Tampa General Hospital, University of Florida, USA

4 Chief of Cardiothoracic Surgery, University of Toledo, Ohio, USA

*Address all correspondence to: jacob.samuel@mayo.edu

References

[1] Maron BJ, Towbin JA, Thiene G, et al. Contemporary definitions and classification of the cardiomyopathies: An American Heart Association scientific statement from the council on clinical cardiology, heart failure and transplantation committee; quality of care and outcomes research and functional genomics and translational biology interdisciplinary working groups; and council on epidemiology and prevention. Circulation. 2006;**113**:1807

[2] Elliott P, Andersson B, Arbustini E, et al. Classification of the cardio-myopathies: A position statement from the European Society of Cardiology working group on myocardial and pericardial diseases. European Heart Journal. 2008;**29**:270

[3] Felker GM, Shaw LK, O'Connor CM. A standardized definition of ischemic cardiomyopathy for use in clinical research. Journal of the American College of Cardiology. 2002;**39**:210-218

[4] Khan MA, Hashim MJ, Mustafa H, Baniyas MY, Al Suwaidi S, AlKatheeri R, et al. Global epidemiology of ischemic heart disease: Results from the global burden of disease study. Cureus. 2020;**12**:e9349

[5] Virani SS, Alonso A, Aparicio HJ, Benjamin EJ, Bittencourt MS, Callaway CW, et al. Heart disease and stroke statistics–2021 update: A report from the American Heart Association. Circulation. 2021;**143**:e254-e743

[6] Elgendy IY, Mahtta D, Pepine CJ. Medical therapy for heart failure caused by ischemic heart disease. Circulation Research. 2019;**124**:1520-1535

[7] Heidenreich PA, Albert NM, Allen LA, Bluemke DA, Butler J, Fonarow GC, et al. Forecasting the impact of heart failure in the United States: A policy statement from the American Heart Association. Circulation. Heart Failure. 2013;**6**:606-619

[8] Yancy CW, Jessup M, Bozkurt B, Butler J, Casey DE Jr, Drazner MH, et al. 2013 ACCF/AHA guideline for the management of heart failure: A report of the American College of Cardiology Foundation/American Heart Association task force on practice guidelines. Journal of the American College of Cardiology. 2013;**62**:e147-e239

[9] Khera S, Panza JA. Surgical revascularization for ischemic cardiomyopathy in the post-STICH era. Cardiology in Review. 2015;**23**(4):153-160. DOI: 10.1097/CRD.0000000000000061 PMID: 25715329

[10] Heusch G, Schulz R. Characterization of hibernating and stunned myocardium. European Heart Journal. 1997;**18**(suppl D):D102-D110

[11] Armstrong WF. "Hibernating" myocardium: Asleep or part dead? Journal of the American College of Cardiology. 1996;**28**:530-535

[12] Wijns W, Vatner SF, Camici PG. Hibernating myocardium. The New England Journal of Medicine. 1998;**339**:173-181

[13] Schuster A, Morton G, Chiribiri A, et al. Imaging in the management of ischemic cardiomyopathy: Special focus on magnetic resonance. Journal of the American College of Cardiology. 2012;**59**:359-370

[14] Rahimtoola SH. A perspective on the three large multicenter randomized clinical trials of coronary bypass surgery for chronic stable angina. Circulation. 1985;**72**(6 Pt 2):V123-V135

[15] Braunwald E, Rutherford JD. Reversible ischemic left ventricular dysfunction: Evidence for the "hibernating myocardium". Journal of the American College of Cardiology. 1986;**8**:1467-1470

[16] Heusch G, Schulz R, Rahimtoola SH. Myocardial hibernation: A delicate balance. American Journal of Physiology. Heart and Circulatory Physiology. 2005;**288**:H984-H999

[17] Rahimtoola SH. The hibernating myocardium. American Heart Journal. 1989;**117**:211-221

[18] Vanoverschelde JL, Wijns W, Borgers M, et al. Chronic myocardial hibernation in humans. From bedside to bench. Circulation. 1997;**95**:1961-1971

[19] Gerber BL, Vanoverschelde JL, Bol A, et al. Myocardial blood flow, glucose uptake, and recruitment of inotropic reserve in chronic left ventricular ischemic dysfunction. Implications for the pathophysiology of chronic myocardial hibernation. Circulation. 1996;**94**:651-659

[20] Depré C, Vanoverschelde JL, Melin JA, et al. Structural and metabolic correlates of the reversibility of chronic left ventricular ischemic dysfunction in humans. The American Journal of Physiology. 1995;**268**(3 Pt 2):H1265-H1275

[21] Im DJ, Youn JC, Lee HJ, Nam K, Suh YJ, Hong YJ, et al. Role of cardiac computed tomography for Etiology evaluation of newly diagnosed heart failure with reduced ejection fraction. Journal of Clinical Medicine. 2020;**9**(7):2270. DOI: 10.3390/jcm9072270

[22] Gatti M, Carisio A, D'Angelo T, Darvizeh F, Dell'Aversana S, Tore D, et al. Cardiovascular magnetic resonance in myocardial infarction with non-obstructive coronary arteries patients: A review. World Journal of Cardiology. 2020;**12**(6):248-261

[23] Subramanyam P, Palaniswamy SS. Does myocardial viability detection improve using a novel combined 99mTc sestamibi infusion and low dose dobutamine infusion in high risk ischemic cardiomyopathy patients? Anatolian Journal of Cardiology. 2020;**24**(2):83-91

[24] Garrett HE, Dennis EW, DeBakey ME. Aortocoronary bypass with saphenous vein graft. Seven-year follow-up. Journal of the American Medical Association. 1973;**223**:792-794

[25] Sabiston DC Jr, The WF, Rienhoff J, lecture. The coronary circulation. The Johns Hopkins Medical Journal. 1974;**134**:314-329

[26] Noon GP. Evolution of surgical treatment of coronary artery occlusive disease. Journal of the American Medical Association. 2009;**301**:970-971

[27] Bakaeen FG, Gaudino M, Whitman G, Doenst T, Ruel M, Taggart DP, et al. 2021: The American Association for Thoracic Surgery expert consensus document: Coronary artery bypass grafting in patients with ischemic cardiomyopathy and heart failure. The Journal of Thoracic and Cardiovascular Surgery. 2021;**162**(3):829-850.e1. DOI: 10.1016/j.jtcvs.2021.04.052

[28] Velazquez EJ, Lee KL, Deja MA, et al. Coronary-artery bypass surgery in patients with left ventricular dysfunction. The New England Journal of Medicine. 2011;**364**(17):1607-1616

[29] Alderman EL, Fisher LD, Litwin P, et al. Results of coronary artery surgery in patients with poor left ventricular function (CASS). Circulation. 1983;**68**:785-795

[30] O'Connor CM, Velazquez EJ, Gardner LH, et al. Comparison of coronary artery bypass grafting versus medical therapy on long-term outcome in patients with ischemic cardiomyopathy (a 25-year experience from the Duke cardiovascular disease databank). The American Journal of Cardiology. 2002;**90**:101-107

[31] Mark DB, Knight JD, Velazquez EJ, Wasilewski J, Howlett JG, Smith PK, et al. Quality-of-life outcomes with coronary artery bypass graft surgery in ischemic left ventricular dysfunction: A randomized trial. Annals of Internal Medicine. 2014;**161**(6):392-399. DOI: 10.7326/M13-1380

[32] Velazquez EJ, Lee KL, Jones RH, Al-Khalidi HR, Hill JA, Panza JA, et al. Coronary-artery bypass surgery in patients with ischemic cardiomyopathy. The New England Journal of Medicine. 2016;**21**(374):1511-1520

[33] Sun LY, Gaudino M, Chen RJ, Bader Eddeen A, Ruel M. Long-term outcomes in patients with severely reduced left ventricular ejection fraction undergoing percutaneous coronary intervention vs coronary artery bypass grafting. JAMA Cardiology. 2020;**5**:631-641

[34] Allman KC, Shaw LJ, Hachamovitch R, Udelson JE. Myocardial viability testing and impact of revascularization on prognosis in patients with coronary artery disease and left ventricular dysfunction: A meta-analysis. Journal of the American College of Cardiology. 2002;**39**(7):1151-1158. DOI: 10.1016/s0735-1097(02)01726-6 PMID: 11923039

[35] Bax JJ, van der Wall EE, Harbinson M. Radionuclide techniques for the assessment of myocardial viability and hibernation. Heart. 2004;**90** (Suppl. 5):v26-v33

[36] Panza JA, Ellis AM, Al-Khalidi HR, Holly TA, Berman DS, Oh JK, et al. Myocardial viability and long-term outcomes in ischemic cardiomyopathy. The New England Journal of Medicine. 2019;**381**(8):739-748

[37] Shah DJ, Kim HW, James O, Parker M, Wu E, Bonow RO, et al. Prevalence of regional myocardial thinning and relationship with myocardial scarring in patients with coronary artery disease. Journal of the American Medical Association. 2013;**309**(9):909-918

[38] Schinkel AF, Poldermans D, Rizzello V, Vanoverschelde JL, Elhendy A, Boersma E, et al. Why do patients with ischemiccardiomyopathyandasubstantial amount of viable myocardium not always recover in function after revascularization? The Journal of Thoracic and Cardiovascular Surgery. 2004;**127**(2):385-390

[39] Bangalore S, Guo Y, Samadashvili Z, Blecker S, Hannan EL. Revascularization in patients with multivessel coronary artery disease and severe left ventricular systolic dysfunction: Everolimus-eluting stents versus coronary artery bypass graft surgery. Circulation. 2016;**133**(22):2132-2140

[40] Sedlis SP, Ramanathan KB, Morrison DA, Sethi G, Sacks J, Henderson W, et al. Outcome of percutaneous coronary intervention versus coronary bypass grafting for patients with low left ventricular ejection fractions, unstable angina pectoris, and risk factors for adverse outcomes with bypass (the AWESOME randomized trial

and registry). The American Journal of Cardiology. 2004;**94**(1):118-120

[41] Carson P, Wertheimer J, Miller A, O'Connor CM, Pina IL, Selzman C, et al. The STICH trial (surgical treatment for ischemic heart failure): Mode-of death results. JACC: Heart Failure. 2013;**1**:308-314

[42] Fallavollita JA, Dare JD, Carter RL, Baldwa S, Canty JM Jr. Denervated myocardium is preferentially associated with sudden cardiac arrest in ischemic cardiomyopathy: A pilot competing risks analysis of cause-specific mortality. Circulation. Cardiovascular Imaging. 2017;**10**(8):e006446

[43] Fallavollita JA, Heavey BM, Luisi AJ Jr, Michalek SM, Baldwa S, Mashtare TL Jr, et al. Regional myocardial sympathetic denervation predicts the risk of sudden cardiac arrest in ischemic cardiomyopathy. Journal of the American College of Cardiology. 2014;**63**:141-149

[44] Vickneson K, Chan SP, Li Y, Bin Abdul Aziz MN, Luo HD, Kang GS, et al. Coronary artery bypass grafting in patients with low ejection fraction: What are the risk factors? The Journal of Cardiovascular Surgery. 2019;**60**:396-405

[45] Kusu-Orkar TE, Kermali M, Oguamanam N, Bithas C, Harky A. Coronary artery bypass grafting: Factors affecting outcomes. Journal of Cardiac Surgery. 2020;**35**:3503-3511

[46] O'Brien SM, Feng L, He X, Xian Y, Jacobs JP, Badhwar V, et al. The Society of Thoracic Surgeons 2018 adult cardiac surgery risk models: Part 2—Statistical methods and results. The Annals of Thoracic Surgery. 2018;**105**:1419-1428

[47] Pichette M, Liszkowski M, Ducharme A. Preoperative optimization of the heart failure patient undergoing cardiac surgery. The Canadian Journal of Cardiology. 2017;**33**:72-79

[48] Christenson JT, Schmuziger M, Simonet F. Effective surgical management of high-risk coronary patients using preoperative intra-aortic balloon counterpulsation therapy. Cardiovascular Surgery. 2001;**9**:383-390

[49] Sa MP, Ferraz PE, Escobar RR, Martins WN, Nunes EO, Vasconcelos FP, et al. Prophylactic intra-aortic balloon pump in high-risk patients undergoing coronary artery bypass surgery: A meta-analysis of randomized controlled trials. Coronary Artery Disease. 2012;**23**:480-486

[50] Pilarczyk K, Boening A, Jakob H, Langebartels G, Markewitz A, Haake N, et al. Preoperative intra-aortic counterpulsation in high-risk patients undergoing cardiac surgery: A meta-analysis of randomized controlled trialsdagger. European Journal of Cardio-Thoracic Surgery. 2016;**49**:5-17

[51] Ramzy D, Soltesz E, Anderson M. New surgical circulatory support system outcomes. ASAIO Journal. 2020;**66**:746-752

[52] Silvestri ERG, Pino JE, Donath E, et al. Impella to unload the left ventricle in patients undergoing venoarterial extracorporeal membrane oxygenation for cardiogenic shock: A systematic review and meta-analysis. Journal of Cardiac Surgery. 2020;**35**:1237-1242

[53] Rihal CS, Naidu SS, Givertz MM, et al. 2015 SCAI/ACC/HFSA/STS clinical expert consensus statement on the use of percutaneous mechanical circulatory support devices in cardiovascular care: Endorsed by the American Heart Association, the Cardiological Society of India, and Sociedad Latino Americana de Cardiologia Intervencion; affirmation

of value by the Canadian Association of Interventional Cardiology-Association Canadienne de Cardiologie d'intervention. Journal of the American College of Cardiology. 2015;**65**:e7-e26

[54] Robinson NB, Audisio K, Bakaeen FG, Gaudino M. Coronary artery bypass grafting in low ejection fraction: State of the art. Current Opinion in Cardiology. 2021;**36**(6):740-747

[55] Bakaeen FG, Shroyer AL, Gammie JS, Sabik JF, Cornwell LD, Coselli JS, et al. Trends in use of off-pump coronary artery bypass grafting: Results from the Society of Thoracic Surgeons adult cardiac surgery database. The Journal of Thoracic and Cardiovascular Surgery. 2014;**148**(856-63):864.e1 discussion 863-4

[56] Bakaeen FG, Gaudino M, Whitman G, Doenst T, Ruel M, Taggart DP, et al. The American Association for Thoracic Surgery expert consensus document: Coronary artery bypass grafting in patients with ischemic cardiomyopathy and heart failure. The Journal of Thoracic and Cardiovascular Surgery. 2021, 2021;**162**(3):829-850.e1

[57] Zeng J, He W, Qu Z, Tang Y, Zhou Q, Zhang B. Cold blood versus crystalloid cardioplegia for myocardial protection in adult cardiac surgery: A meta-analysis of randomized controlled studies. Journal of Cardiothoracic and Vascular Anesthesia. 2014;**28**:674-681

[58] Fan Y, Zhang AM, Xiao YB, Weng YG, Hetzer R. Warm versus cold cardioplegia for heart surgery: A meta-analysis. European Journal of Cardio-Thoracic Surgery. 2010;**37**:912-919

[59] Gambardella I, Gaudino MFL, Antoniou GA, Rahouma M, Worku B, Tranbaugh RF, et al. Single- versus multidose cardioplegia in adult cardiac surgery patients: A meta-analysis. The Journal of Thoracic and Cardiovascular Surgery. 2020;**160**:1195-202.e12

[60] Oriaku G, Xiang B, Dai G, Shen J, Sun J, Lindsay WG, et al. Effects of retrograde cardioplegia on myocardial perfusion and energy metabolism in immature porcine myocardium. The Journal of Thoracic and Cardiovascular Surgery. 2000;**119**:1102-1109

[61] Siddiqi S, Blackstone EH, Bakaeen FG. Bretschneider and del Nido solutions: Are they safe for coronary artery bypass grafting? If so, how should we use them? Journal of Cardiac Surgery. 2018;**33**:229-234

[62] Borger MA, Rao V, Weisel RD, Floh AA, Cohen G, Feindel CM, et al. Reoperative coronary bypass surgery: Effect of patent grafts and retrograde cardioplegia. The Journal of Thoracic and Cardiovascular Surgery. 2001;**121**:83-90

[63] Puskas JD, Gaudino M, Taggart DP. Experience is crucial in off-pump coronary artery bypass grafting. Circulation. 2019;**139**:1872-1875

[64] Jarral OA, Saso S, Athanasiou T. Off-pump coronary artery bypass in patients with left ventricular dysfunction: A meta-analysis. The Annals of Thoracic Surgery. 2011;**92**:1686-1694

[65] Guan Z, Guan X, Gu K, Lin X, Lin J, Zhou W, et al. Short-term outcomes of on vs off-pump coronary artery bypass grafting in patients with left ventricular dysfunction: A systematic review and meta-analysis. Journal of Cardiothoracic Surgery. 2020;**15**:84

[66] Ueki C, Miyata H, Motomura N, Sakaguchi G, Akimoto T, Takamoto S. Off pump versus on-pump coronary artery bypass grafting in patients with left ventricular dysfunction. The Journal

of Thoracic and Cardiovascular Surgery. 2016;**151**:1092-1098

[67] Al Jaaly E, Chaudhry UA, Harling L, Athanasiou T. Should we consider beating-heart on-pump coronary artery bypass grafting over conventional cardioplegic arrest to improve postoperative outcomes in selected patients? Interactive Cardiovascular and Thoracic Surgery. 2015;**20**:538-545

[68] Pegg TJ, Selvanayagam JB, Francis JM, Karamitsos TD, Maunsell Z, Yu LM, et al. A randomized trial of on-pump beating heart and conventional cardioplegic arrest in coronary artery bypass surgery patients with impaired left ventricular function using cardiac magnetic resonance imaging and biochemical markers. Circulation. 2008;**118**:2130-2138

[69] Aldea GS, Bakaeen FG, Pal J, Fremes S, Head SJ, Sabik J, et al. The Society of Thoracic Surgeons clinical practice guidelines on arterial conduits for coronary artery bypass grafting. The Annals of Thoracic Surgery. 2016;**101**:801-809

[70] Neumann FJ, Sousa-Uva M, Ahlsson A, Alfonso F, Banning AP, Benedetto U, et al. 2018 ESC/EACTS guidelines on myocardial revascularization. European Heart Journal. 2019;**40**:87-165

[71] Gaudino M, Benedetto U, Taggart DP. Radial-artery grafts for coronary-artery bypass surgery. The New England Journal of Medicine. 2018;**379**:1967-1968

[72] Pu A, Ding L, Shin J, Price J, Skarsgard P, Wong DR, et al. Long-term outcomes of multiple arterial coronary artery bypass grafting: A population-based study of patients in British Columbia, Canada. JAMA Cardiology. 2017;**2**:1187-1196

[73] Weiss AJ, Zhao S, Tian DH, Taggart DP, Yan TD. A meta-analysis comparing bilateral internal mammary artery with left internal mammary artery for coronary artery bypass grafting. Annals of Cardiothoracic Surgery. 2013;**2**:390-400

[74] Shahian DM, O'Brien SM, Filardo G, Ferraris VA, Haan CK, Rich JB, et al. The Society of Thoracic Surgeons 2008 cardiac surgery risk models: Part 1—Coronary artery bypass grafting surgery. The Annals of Thoracic Surgery. 2009;**88**:S2-S22

[75] He GW, Taggart DP. Spasm in arterial grafts in coronary artery bypass grafting surgery. The Annals of Thoracic Surgery. 2016;**101**:1222-1229

[76] Silva M, Rong LQ, Naik A, Rahouma M, Hameed I, Robinson B, et al. Intraoperative graft flow profiles in coronary artery bypass surgery: A metaanalysis. Journal of Cardiac Surgery. 2020;**35**:279-285

[77] Jones EL, Lattouf OM, Weintraub WS. Catastrophic consequences of internal mammary artery hypoperfusion. The Journal of Thoracic and Cardiovascular Surgery. 1989;**98**:902-907

[78] Navia D, Cosgrove DM III, Lytle BW, Taylor PC, McCarthy PM, Stewart RW, et al. Is the internal thoracic artery the conduit of choice to replace a stenotic vein graft? The Annals of Thoracic Surgery. 1994;**57**:40-44

[79] Gaudino M, Benedetto U, Fremes S, Biondi-Zoccai G, Sedrakyan A, Puskas JD, et al. Radial-artery or saphenous-vein grafts in coronary-artery bypass surgery. The New England Journal of Medicine. 2018;**378**:2069-2077

[80] Lytle BW, Blackstone EH, Sabik JF, Houghtaling P, Loop FD, Cosgrove DM.

The effect of bilateral internal thoracic artery grafting on survival during 20 postoperative years. The Annals of Thoracic Surgery. 2004;**78**:2005-2014

[81] Schwann TA, Al-Shaar L, Tranbaugh RF, Dimitrova KR, Hoffman DM, Geller CM, et al. Multi versus single arterial coronary bypass graft surgery across the ejection fraction spectrum. The Annals of Thoracic Surgery. 2015;**100**:810-818

[82] Samadashvili Z, Sundt TM III, Wechsler A, Chikwe J, Adams DH, Smith CR, et al. Multiple versus single arterial coronary bypass graft surgery for multivessel disease. Journal of the American College of Cardiology. 2019;**74**:1275-1285

[83] Chikwe J, Sun E, Hannan EL, Itagaki S, Lee T, Adams DH, et al. Outcomes of second arterial conduits in patients undergoing multivessel coronary artery bypass graft surgery. Journal of the American College of Cardiology. 2019;**74**:2238-2248

[84] Mohammadi S, Kalavrouziotis D, Cresce G, Dagenais F, Dumont E, Charbonneau E, et al. Bilateral internal thoracic artery use in patients with low ejection fraction: Is there any additional long-term benefit? European Journal of Cardio-Thoracic Surgery. 2014;**46**:425-431

[85] Gaudino M, Bakaeen F, Benedetto U, Rahouma M, Di Franco A, Tam DY, et al. Use rate and outcome in bilateral internal thoracic artery grafting: Insights from a systematic review and meta-analysis. Journal of the American Heart Association. 2018;**7**:e009361

[86] Benedetto U, CodispotiM. Age cutoff for the loss of survival benefit from use of radial artery in coronary artery bypass grafting. The Journal of Thoracic and Cardiovascular Surgery. 2013;**146**:1078-1085

[87] Benedetto U, Amrani M, Raja SG. Guidance for the use of bilateral internal thoracic arteries according to survival benefit across age groups. The Journal of Thoracic and Cardiovascular Surgery. 2014;**148**:2706-2711

[88] Gaudino M, Samadashvili Z, Hameed I, Chikwe J, Girardi LN, Hannan EL. Differences in long-term outcomes after coronary artery bypass grafting using single vs multiple arterial grafts and the association with sex. JAMA Cardiology. 2020;**6**:401-409

[89] Ad N, Barnett SD, Haan CK, et al. Does preoperative atrial fibrillation increase the risk for mortality and morbidity after coronary artery bypass grafting? The Journal of Thoracic and Cardiovascular Surgery. 2009;**137**:901-906

[90] Badhwar V, Rankin JS, Damiano RJ, et al. The Society of Thoracic Surgeons 2017 clinical practice guidelines for the surgical treatment of atrial fibrillation. The Annals of Thoracic Surgery. 2017;**103**:329-341

[91] Hindricks G, Potpara T, Dagres N, et al. 2020 ESC guidelines for the diagnosis and management of atrial fibrillation developed in collaboration with the European Association for Cardio-Thoracic Surgery (EACTS). European Heart Journal. 2021;**42**:373-498

[92] Malaisrie SC, McCarthy PM, Kruse J, et al. Ablation of atrial fibrillation during coronary artery bypass grafting: Late outcomes in a Medicare population. The Journal of Thoracic and Cardiovascular Surgery. 2019;**161**:1251.e1-1261.e1

[93] Guglin M, Chen R, Curtis AB. Sinus rhythm is associated with fewer heart failure symptoms: Insights from

the AFFIRM trial. Heart Rhythm. 2010;7:596-601

[94] Ad N, Henry L, Hunt S. The impact of surgical ablation in patients with low ejection fraction, heart failure, and atrial fibrillation. European Journal of Cardio-Thoracic Surgery. 2011;**40**:70-76

[95] Pecha S, Ahmadzade T, Schafer T, et al. Safety and feasibility of concomitant surgical ablation of atrial fibrillation in patients with severely reduced left ventricular ejection fraction. European Journal of Cardio-Thoracic Surgery. 2014;**46**:67-71

[96] Goliasch G, Bartko PE, Pavo N, et al. Refining the prognostic impact of functional mitral regurgitation in chronic heart failure. European Heart Journal. 2018;**39**:39-46

[97] Michler RE, Smith PK, Parides MK, Ailawadi G, Thourani V, Moskowitz AJ, et al. Two-year outcomes of surgical treatment of moderate ischemic mitral regurgitation. The New England Journal of Medicine. 2016;**374**:1932-1941

[98] Chan KM, Punjabi PP, Flather M, Wage R, Symmonds K, Roussin I, et al. Coronary artery bypass surgery with or without mitral valve annuloplasty in moderate functional ischemic mitral regurgitation: Final results of the randomized ischemic mitral evaluation (RIME) trial. Circulation. 2012;**126**:2502-2510

[99] Fattouch K, Guccione F, Sampognaro R, Panzarella G, Corrado E, Navarra E, et al. POINT: Efficacy of adding mitral valve restrictive annuloplasty to coronary artery bypass grafting in patients with moderate ischemic mitral valve regurgitation: A randomized trial. The Journal of Thoracic and Cardiovascular Surgery. 2009;**138**:278-285

[100] Goldstein D, Moskowitz AJ, Gelijns AC, Ailawadi G, Parides MK, Perrault LP, et al. Two-year outcomes of surgical treatment of severe ischemic mitral regurgitation. The New England Journal of Medicine. 2016;**374**:344-353

[101] Nappi F, Lusini M, Spadaccio C, Nenna A, Covino E, Acar C, et al. Papillary muscle approximation versus restrictive annuloplasty alone for severe ischemic mitral regurgitation. Journal of the American College of Cardiology. 2016;**67**:2334-2346

[102] Fattouch K, Lancellotti P, Castrovinci S, Murana G, Sampognaro R, Corrado E, et al. Papillary muscle relocation in conjunction with valve annuloplasty improve repair results in severe ischemic mitral regurgitation. The Journal of Thoracic and Cardiovascular Surgery. 2012;**143**:1352-1355

[103] Malhotra A, Sharma P, Garg P, Bishnoi A, Kothari J, Pujara J. Ring annuloplasty for ischemic mitral regurgitation: A single center experience. Asian Cardiovascular & Thoracic Annals. 2014;**22**(7):781-786

[104] Haywood N, Mehaffey JH, Chancellor WZ, Beller JP, Speir A, Quader M, et al. Burden of tricuspid regurgitation in patients undergoing coronary artery bypass grafting. The Annals of Thoracic Surgery. 2021;**111**:44-50

[105] Bertrand PB, Overbey JR, Zeng X, Levine RA, Ailawadi G, Acker MA, et al. Progression of tricuspid regurgitation after surgery for ischemic mitral regurgitation. Journal of the American College of Cardiology. 2021;**77**:713-724

[106] Otto CM, Nishimura RA, Bonow RO, Carabello BA, Erwin JP III, Gentile F, et al. 2020 ACC/AHA

guideline for the management of patients with valvular heart disease: A report of the American College of Cardiology/ American Heart Association joint committee on clinical practice guidelines. Journal of the American College of Cardiology. 2021;77:e25-e197

[107] Buckberg G, Athanasuleas C, Conte J. Surgical ventricular restoration for the treatment of heart failure. Nature Reviews. Cardiology. 2012;**9**:703-716

[108] O'Neill JO, Starling RC, McCarthy PM, Albert NM, Lytle BW, Navia J, et al. The impact of left ventricular reconstruction on survival in patients with ischemic cardiomyopathy. European Journal of Cardio-Thoracic Surgery. 2006;**30**:753-759

[109] Ribeiro GA, da Costa CE, Lopes MM, et al. Left ventricular reconstruction benefits patients with ischemic cardiomyopathy and nonviable myocardium. European Journal of Cardio-Thoracic Surgery. 2006;**29**:196-201

[110] Prucz RB, Weiss ES, Patel ND, et al. Coronary artery bypass grafting with or without surgical ventricular restoration: A comparison. The Annals of Thoracic Surgery. 2008;**86**:806-814

[111] Jones RH, Velazquez EJ, Michler RE, Sopko G, Oh JK, O'Connor CM, et al. Coronary bypass surgery with or without surgical ventricular reconstruction. The New England Journal of Medicine. 2009;**360**:1705-1717

[112] Buckberg GD, Athanasuleas CL, Wechsler AS, Beyersdorf F, Conte JV, Strobeck JE. The STICH trial unravelled. European Journal of Heart Failure. 2010;**12**:1024-1027

[113] Isomura T, Hoshino J, Fukada Y, Kitamura A, Katahira S, Kondo T, et al. Volume reduction rate by surgical ventricular restoration determines late outcome in ischaemic cardiomyopathy. European Journal of Heart Failure. 2011;**13**:423-431

[114] Di Donato M, Castelvecchio S, Menicanti L. End-systolic volume following surgical ventricular reconstruction impacts survival in patients with ischaemic dilated cardiomyopathy. European Journal of Heart Failure. 2010;**12**:375-381

[115] Antman EM, Anbe DT, Armstrong PW, Bates ER, Green LA, Hand M, et al. ACC/AHA guidelines for the management of patients with ST-elevation myocardial infarction—Executive summary: A report of the American College of Cardiology/ American Heart Association task force on practice guidelines (writing committee to revise the 1999 guidelines for the management of patients with acute myocardial infarction). [published correction appears in circulation. 2005;111:2013]. Circulation. 2004;**110**:588-636

[116] Morici N, Oliva F, Ajello S, Stucchi M, Sacco A, Cipriani MG, et al. Management of cardiogenic shock in acute decompensated chronic heart failure: The ALTSHOCK phase II clinical trial. American Heart Journal. 2018;**204**:196-201

[117] McGee MG, Zillgitt SL, Trono R, Turner SA, Davis GL, Fuqua JM, et al. Retrospective analyses of the need for mechanical circulatory support (intraaortic balloon pump/abdominal left ventricular assist device or partial artificial heart) after cardiopulmonary bypass. A 44 month study of 14,168 patients. The American Journal of Cardiology. 1980;**46**:135-142

[118] Boeken U, Feindt P, Litmathe J, Kurt M, Gams E. Intraaortic balloon

pumping in patients with right ventricular insufficiency after cardiac surgery: Parameters to predict failure of IABP support. The Thoracic and Cardiovascular Surgeon. 2009;**57**:324-328

[119] Engstrom AE, Granfeldt H, Seybold-Epting W, Dahm M, Cocchieri R, Driessen AH, et al. Mechanical circulatory support with the Impella 5.0 device for postcardiotomy cardiogenic shock: A three-center experience. Minerva Cardioangiologica. 2013;**61**:539-546

[120] David CH, Quessard A, Mastroianni C, Hekimian G, Amour J, Leprince P, et al. Mechanical circulatory support with the Impella 5.0 and the Impella left direct pumps for postcardiotomy cardiogenic shock at La Pitie-Salpetriere hospital. European Journal of Cardio-Thoracic Surgery. 2020;**57**:183-188

[121] Griffith BP, Anderson MB, Samuels LE, Pae WE Jr, Naka Y, Frazier OH. The RECOVER I: A multicenter prospective study of Impella 5.0/LD for postcardiotomy circulatory support. The Journal of Thoracic and Cardiovascular Surgery. 2013;**145**:548-554

[122] Lorusso R, Whitman G, MilojevicM RG, McMullan DM, Boeken U, et al. EACTS/ELSO/STS/AATS expert consensus on post-cardiotomy extracorporeal life support in adult patients. The Journal of Thoracic and Cardiovascular Surgery. 2020;**2021**(161):1287-1331

[123] Rastan AJ, Dege A, Mohr M, Doll N, Falk V, Walther T, et al. Early and late outcomes of 517 consecutive adult patients treated with extracorporeal membrane oxygenation for refractory postcardiotomy cardiogenic shock. The Journal of Thoracic and Cardiovascular Surgery. 2010;**139**:302-311

[124] Elsharkawy HA, Li L, Esa WA, Sessler DI, Bashour CA. Outcome in patients who require venoarterial extracorporeal membrane oxygenation support after cardiac surgery. Journal of Cardiothoracic and Vascular Anesthesia. 2010;**24**:946-951

[125] Wang L, Wang H, Hou X. Clinical outcomes of adult patients who receive extracorporeal membrane oxygenation for postcardiotomy cardiogenic shock: A systematic review and meta-analysis. Journal of Cardiothoracic and Vascular Anesthesia. 2018;**32**:2087-2093

[126] Mariscalco G, Salsano A, Fiore A, Dalen M, Ruggieri VG, Saeed D, et al. Peripheral versus central extracorporeal membrane oxygenation for postcardiotomy shock: Multicenter registry, systematic review, and meta-analysis. The Journal of Thoracic and Cardiovascular Surgery. 2020;**160**: 1207-1216

[127] Schrage B, Becher PM, Bernhardt A, Bezerra H, Blankenberg S, Brunner S, et al. Left ventricular unloading is associated with lower mortality in patients with cardiogenic shock treated with venoarterial extracorporeal membrane oxygenation: Results from an international, multicenter cohort study. Circulation. 2020;**142**:2095-2106

[128] Russo JJ, Aleksova N, Pitcher I, Couture E, Parlow S, Faraz M, et al. Left ventricular- unloading during extracorporeal membrane oxygenation in patients with cardiogenic shock. Journal of the American College of Cardiology. 2019;**73**:654-662

[129] Murphy SP, Ibrahim NE, Januzzi JL Jr. Heart failure with reduced ejection fraction: A review. Journal of the American Medical Association. 2020;**324**:488-504

[130] Maddox TM, Januzzi JL Jr, Allen LA, Breathett K, Butler J, Davis LL, et al. 2021 update to the 2017 ACC expert consensus decision pathway for optimization of heart failure treatment: Answers to 10 pivotal issues about heart failure with reduced ejection fraction: A report of the American College of Cardiology solution set oversight committee. Journal of the American College of Cardiology. 2021;**77**:772-810

[131] Hernandez AF, Greiner MA, Fonarow GC, Hammill BG, Heidenreich PA, Yancy CW, et al. Relationship between early physician follow-up and 30-day readmission among Medicare beneficiaries hospitalized for heart failure. Journal of the American Medical Association. 2010;**303**:1716-1722

[132] Farsky PS, White J, Al-Khalidi HR, Sueta CA, Rouleau JL, Panza JA, et al. O'Connor CM; working group and surgical treatment for IsChemic heart failure trial Investigators. Optimal medical therapy with or without surgical revascularization and long-term outcomes in ischemic cardiomyopathy. The Journal of Thoracic and Cardiovascular Surgery. 2021;**S0022-5223**(20):33449-33448

Section 3

CABG versus PCI

Chapter 7

Is Coronary Artery Bypass Grafting (CABG) Surgery Still Preferable to Percutaneous Coronary Intervention (PCI) in View of Long-Term Outcomes among Diabetic Patients?

Ahmad Farouk Musa

Abstract

Coronary Artery Bypass Grafting (CABG) is the preferred revascularization modality among diabetic patients due to extensive coronary involvement and elevated risk of restenosis. Since drug-eluting stent significantly reduces restenosis, we expect it to narrow down the long-term benefit-gap between these two revascularization strategies. In our review, we compare the long-term outcomes of Percutaneous Coronary Intervention (PCI) to CABG in diabetic patients. While PCI can be a reasonable alternative to CABG at a low SYNTAX (Synergy between Percutaneous Coronary Intervention with Taxus and Cardiac Surgery) score, an intermediate-high SYNTAX score makes CABG necessary. In left main stem occlusion, PCI and CABG demonstrated similar long-term outcomes. However, in cases of bifurcation or unprotected left main stem disease, revascularization is best done via CABG. Indeed, CABG is the main revascularization therapy in multivessel involvement— it lowers the risk of all-cause mortality, myocardial infarction and repeat revascularization at the expense of increasessd stroke. Glycaemic control, use of anti-platelet agents and feelings of disability are all factors that can potentially affect long-term outcomes. We expect hybrid coronary revascularization (HCR) involving both robotic surgery and PCI to be the future trend in treating diabetic patients with multivessel disease, although its clinical use needs further studies.

Keywords: Coronary Artery Bypass Grafting (CABG), Percutaneous Coronary Intervention (PCI), diabetic patients, long-term outcomes, hybrid coronary revascularization (HCR)

1. Introduction

Revascularization is the preferred treatment procedure in patients with coronary artery disease (CAD). Coronary Artery Bypass Grafting (CABG) and Percutaneous

Coronary Intervention (PCI), formerly known as Percutaneous Transluminal Coronary Angioplasty (PTCA), are the two methods of revascularization that are widely performed worldwide. Contrary to CABG, PCI is less invasive. Moreover, it has a shorter procedural time and duration of hospital stay. Nonetheless, it is associated with a higher risk of repeat revascularization.

About 25–30% of patients admitted with acute coronary syndrome (ACS) are reported to have underlying diabetes [1]. Compared to their non-diabetic counterparts, diabetic patients suffer from a significantly higher rate of mortality and adverse events [2–4]. While early revascularization could enhance their prognosis, [5] the long-term merits of utilising either CABG or PCI are yet to be conclusively established.

2. Aim

Our study aims to find out whether diabetic patients have a better long-term prognosis with PCI compared to CABG.

3. Methods

Using PubMed, MEDLINE, Cochrane and Embase database, we conducted a literature search dating from January 2010 to June 2020 to locate relevant articles. We used Medical Subject Heading (MeSH) terms such as "diabetes mellitus", "Percutaneous Transluminal Coronary Angioplasty" and "Coronary Artery Bypass Surgery" to identify journal articles. We also cross-checked references to allow the selection of additional pertinent references.

Studies that were included fall into the following three categories: (1) they were published from January 2010 to June 2020; (2) they had a minimum duration of patient follow-up of five years; and (3) they involved revascularization of patients with Type 2 diabetes mellitus.

Studies that were excluded fall into the following four categories:

1. they were published as editorials, reviews and letters since they were prone to bias;

2. they involved other subtypes of diabetes such as Type 1 diabetes mellitus, Maturity-Onset Diabetes of the Young (MODY), Latent Autoimmune Diabetes of Adulthood (LADA) and impaired glucose tolerance, not to mention prediabetes states with a different mechanism of platelet dysfunction and thrombosis;

3. they are based on revascularization for diseases such as valvular heart disease, cardiogenic shock and arrhythmias, all of which are associated with different risks and complications; and

4. they involved repeat revascularization in patients with a history of CABG and PCI.

Based on the above inclusion and exclusion criteria, data extraction was performed.

The primary endpoints were as follows: mortality rate, risk of myocardial infarction (MI), stroke and repeat revascularization.

4. Results

Regarding left main stem disease (LMSD), both CABG and PTCA arms yielded similar mortality and composite endpoints of all-cause mortality, myocardial infarction (MI) and stroke risk. Additionally, the CABG arm reported a lower risk of target vessel revascularization. **Table 1** below describes the randomized controlled trials and observational studies of PTCA versus CABG that were included in our analyses.

First author Year	**Study design**	**Region**	**PTCA (n) CABG (n)**	**Follow-up**	**All cause-mortality and adverse outcomes**
Left Main Stem Disease (LMSD)					
Yu (2014) [6]	Retrosp-ective study	China	PTCA: 143 CABG: 131 Total: 274	7.1 years	All-cause mortality: Similar in both arms (HR: 0.752, 95% CI 0.380–1.489 $p = 0.413$) Death, myocardial infarction and stroke: Similar in both arms (HR: 0.794, 95% CI: 0.463–1.361 $p = 0.401$) Repeat revascularization: Higher in PTCA arm (HR: 2.112, 95% CI 1.102–4.048 $p = 0.024$)
Lee (2020) [7]	Multicen-tre, non-random-ised trial	Korea	PTCA: 395 CABG: 327 Total:722	12 years	All-cause mortality: Similar in both arms (HR: 1.08, 95% CI 0.85–1.38 $p = 0.54$) Death, Q-wave MI, stroke: similar in both arms (HR: 1.25, 95% CI 0.97–1.61 $p = 0.09$) Repeat revascularization: Higher in PTCA arm (HR: 4.07, 95% CI 2.65–6.26 $p < 0.0001$)
Multivessel disease (MVD)					
Onuma (2010) [8]	Population from ARTS I and ARTS II trial	20 countries	PTCA: 159 CABG: 96 Total:255	5 years	All-cause mortality: Similar in both arms (HR:1.11, 95% CI 0.47–2.66 $p = 0.81$) MI: Similar in both arms (HR:1.19, 95% CI 0.38–3.76 $p = 0.76$) Stroke: Similar in both arms (HR:1.24, 95% CI 0.42–3.65 $p = 0.70$) Repeat revascularization: Lower in CABG arm (HR:0.31, 95% CI 0.16–0.62 $p = 0.001$)

First author Year	Study design	Region	PTCA (n) CABG (n)	Follow-up	All cause-mortality and adverse outcomes
Contini (2012) [9]	Multicen-tre, non-randomi-sed, open label ARTS-II trial	Italy	PTCA: 1466 CABG: 1419 Total:2885	5 years	All-cause mortality: Higher in PTCA arm (HR: 1.8, 95% CI 1.4–2.2 $p < 0.0001$) MI: Higher in PTCA arm (HR: 3.3, 95% CI 2.4–4.6 $p < 0.0001$) Stroke: Similar in both arms (HR: 0.8, 95% CI 0.5–1.2 $p = 0.26$) Repeat revascularization: Higher in PTCA arm (HR: 4.5, 95% CI 3.4–6.1 $p < 0.0001$)
Kim (2012) [10]	Single-centre prospect-ive, non-randomi-sed observant-ional cohort study	Korea	PTCA: 489 CABG: 402 Total:891	5.6 years	All-cause mortality: Similar in both arms (HR 1.01, 95% CI 0.77 to 1.33, $p = 0.96$) Repeat revascularization: Higher in PTCA arm (HR 3.69, 95% CI 2.64 to 5.17, $p < 0.001$)
Moshkovitz (2012) [11]	Retrospe-ctive study	Israel	PTCA: 271 CABG: 226 Total:497	62 months	All-cause mortality: Higher in PTCA arm (HR:3.01, 95% CI 1.59 to 5.73, $p = 0.0001$) Repeat revascularization: Higher in PTCA arm (HR 7.00, 95% CI: 3.1 to 15.70)
Freedom Study (2012) [12]	Multicentre randomised trial	140 internat-ional centers	PTCA: 953 CABG: 947 Total: 1900	2 to 6.75 years	All-cause mortality: Higher in PTCA arm (PTCA 16.3% vs. CABG 10.6%; $p = 0.049$) MI: Higher in PTCA arm (PTCA: 13.9% vs. CABG:6.0%; $p < 0.001$) Stroke: Higher in CABG arm (PTCA:2.4% vs. CABG: 5.2%; $p = 0.03$) Repeat revascularization: Higher in PTCA arm (PTCA: 12.6% vs. CABG: 4.8%; $p < 0.001$)
BEST Trial (2015) [13]	Prospect-ive, open-label, randomi-sed trial	South Korea, China, Malay-sia, Thailand	PTCA: 438 CABG:442 Total: 880	1–5.2 years	All-cause mortality: Similar in both arms (HR: 1.34, 95% CI 0.77–2.34 $p = 0.30$) MI: Similar in both arms (HR: 1.76, 95% CI 0.87–3.58 $p = 0.11$) Stroke: Similar in both arms (HR: 0.86, 95% CI 0.39–1.93 $p = 0.72$) Repeat revascularization: Higher in PTCA arm (HR: 2.09, 95% CI 1.28–3.41 $p = 0.003$)

First author Year	Study design	Region	PTCA (n) CABG (n)	Follow-up	All cause-mortality and adverse outcomes
FREEDOM Follow-on Study (2019) [14]	Multicen-tre randomi-sed trial	25 centers	PTCA:478 CABG:465 Total: 943	7.5 years	All-cause mortality: higher in PTCA arm (PTCA 24.3% vs. CABG 18.3%; HR:1.36; 95% CI: 1.07 to 1.74; $p = 0.01$)
LMSD and/or MVD					
SYNTAX trial (2013) [15]	Prospect-ive multinat-ional randomi-sed trial	Multi-national	PTCA: 897 CABG: 903 Total:1800	5 years	All-cause mortality: Similar in both arms (PTCA: 19.5% vs. CABG: 12.9%; $p = 0.065$) MI: Similar in both arms (PTCA: 9.0% vs. CABG: 5.4%; $p = 0.20$). Stroke: Similar in both arms (PTCA:3.0% vs. CABG: 4.7%; $p = 0.34$) Repeat revascularization: Higher in PTCA arm (PTCA: 35.3% vs. CABG: 14.6%; $p < 0.001$)

LMSD: left main stem disease; MVD: multivessel disease; MI: myocardial infarction, PTCA: percutaneous transluminal coronary angioplasty, CABG: Coronary Artery Bypass Grafting, HR: hazard ratio, Cl: Confidence interval

Table 1.
Randomised controlled trials and observational studies of PTCA vs CABG.

In the case of multivessel disease (MVD), a significantly higher risk of repeat revascularization in patients undergoing PTCA was consistently reported in four observational studies and three randomised controlled trials. On the contrary, data regarding mortality rate, risk of myocardial infarction and stroke were inconsistent. We observed similar findings in Onuma's [8] and Kim's [10] study (Onuma: HR:1.11, 95% CI 0.47–2.66 $p = 0.81$; Kim: HR 1.01, 95% CI 0.77 to 1.33, $p = 0.96$). However, PTCA incurred a higher mortality risk in other studies. One such study is the FREEDOM Follow-On study [14] that reports the survival rate of patients in the FREEDOM trial with an extended follow-up period. The authors Farkouh et al. [14] concluded that only after the second year follow-up did the mortality curves begin to separate; they also noted increasing discrepancy as the follow-up duration was extrapolated.

Meanwhile, the risk of myocardial infarction varied. While similar MI risk was observed in Onuma's study [8] (HR:1.19, 95% CI 0.38–3.76 $p = 0.76$) and BEST Trial [13] (HR: 1.76, 95% CI 0.87–3.58 $p = 0.11$), Contini's [9] (HR: 3.3, 95% CI 2.4–4.6 $p < 0.0001$) and FREEDOM study [12] (PTCA: 13.9% vs. CABG:6.0%; $p < 0.001$) reported a significantly higher risk in the PTCA arm. Likewise, Onuma's [8] (HR:1.24, 95% CI 0.42–3.65 $p = 0.70$), Contini's study [9] (HR: 0.8, 95% CI 0.5–1.2 $p = 0.26$) and BEST Trial [13] (HR: 0.86, 95% CI 0.39–1.93 $p = 0.72$) documented comparable risk of stroke. But this was not the case in FREEDOM study [12] (PTCA:2.4% vs. CABG: 5.2%; $p = 0.03$).

SYNTAX trial [15] compared treatment outcomes of PTCA and CABG in patients with LMS and/or MVD with a follow-up duration of five years. Using Synergy Between Percutaneous Coronary Intervention with Taxus and Cardiac Surgery (SYNTAX) score, subgroup analyses were performed to evaluate the adverse outcomes of each revascularization strategy. In SYNTAX trial, both groups demonstrated

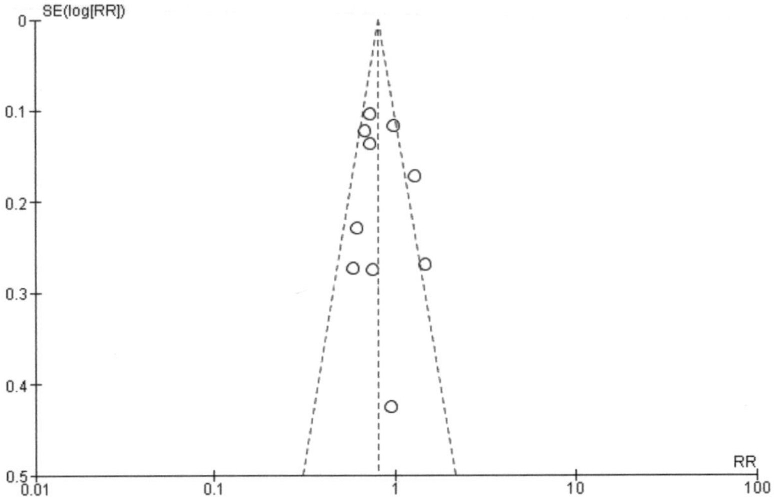

Figure 1.
Funnel plot for assessment of publication bias of observational and randomised trials comparing CABG with PTCA for the endpoint of all-cause mortality. SE: Standard Error. RR: Risk Ratio.

similar survival and other adverse outcomes rates. On the contrary, the PTCA group suffered a higher burden of repeat revascularization.

Referring to **Figure 1**, this study comprised ten studies (observational and randomised trials). It followed the rule of thumb regarding tests for funnel plot asymmetry: a minimum ten studies should be included in the meta-analyses. With fewer studies, the power of the tests is too low to tell apart chance from real asymmetry.

The Funnel Plot displayed a certain heterogeneity; only two studies were outliers. Conversely, Egger's test confirmed the plot asymmetry. (Heterogeneity: ChiSq = 21.60; df = 9; p = 0.01, I^2 = 58%). This is not surprising since both observational and randomised trials were included. Moreover, publication bias cannot be ruled out since the funnel plot might have excluded smaller studies with negative outcomes.

Table 2 refers to one study-level pooled analyses and four meta-analyses which compared the rate of mortality and adverse outcomes of PTCA-DES *vs* CABG in diabetic patients with a minimum five-year follow-up.

Author & Year	Follow up (years)	RCT & OS (n)	Number of patients (n)	All- cause mortality and adverse outcomes
Hakeem (2013) [16]	2–5	RCT: 4 OS:0 Total: 4	PTCA: 1539 CABG:1513 Total: 3052	All- cause mortality: Higher in PTCA arm (PTCA 14% vs. CABG9.7%, RR 1.51, 95% CI 1.09 to 2.10, p = 0.01) MI: Similar in both arms (PTCA 10.3% vs. CABG 5.9%, RR 1.44, 95% CI 0.79 to 2.6, p = 0.23) Stroke: Lower in PTCA arm (PTCA 2.3% vs. CABG 3.8%, RR 0.59, 95% CI 0.39 to 0.90, p = 0.01) Repeat revascularization: Higher in PTCA arm (PTCA 17.4% vs. CABG 8.0%, RR 1.85, 95% CI 1.0 to 3.40, p = 0.05)

Author & Year	Follow up (years)	RCT & OS (n)	Number of patients (n)	All- cause mortality and adverse outcomes
Verma (2013) [17]	5 years	RCT: 8 OS: 0 Total: 8	Total: 3612	All- cause mortality: Lower in CABG arm (RR 0·67, 95% CI 0·52–0·86; p = 0·002) MI: Similar in both arms (RR 0·76, 95% CI 0·44–1·29; p = 0·30) Stroke: Higher in CABG arm (RR 2·41, 95% CI 1·22–4·76; p = 0·01) Repeat revascularization: Lower in CABG arm (RR 0.41, 95% CI 0·29–0·59; p < 0·0001)
Luca (2014) [18]	1–5	RCT: 4 OS:10 Total: 14	PTCA: 3650 CABG: 3422 Total: 7072	All- cause mortality: Lower in CABG arm (CABG 7.3% vs. PTCA 10.4%, 95%CI: 0.65 (0.55–0.77), p < 0.0001; p_{het} = 0.00001) Stroke: Higher in CABG arm (CABG 3.6% vs. PTCA 1.4%, 95%CI: 2.34 (1.63–3.35), p < 0.00001, p_{het} = 0.71). Repeat revascularization: Lower in CABG arm (CABG 5.2% vs. PTCA 15.7%, 95% CI: 0.30 (0.25–0.36), p < 0.00001, p_{het} = 0.02)
Huang (2015) [19]	1–5.1	RCT: 4 OS: 15 Total: 19	PTCA: 4502 CABG:4363 Total: 8865	All-cause mortality: Similar in both arms (PTCA 11.7% vs. CABG 9.1%, RR 1.23, 95% CI 1.00–1.53, p = 0.06). MI: Higher in PTCA arm (PTCA 8.5% vs. CABG 4.6%, RR 1.68, 95% CI 1.20–2.37, p = 0.003) Stroke: Lower in PTCA arm (PTCA 2.0% vs. CABG 3.9%, RR 0.51, 95% CI 0.39–0.67, p < 0.00001) Repeat revascularization: Higher in PTCA arm (PTCA 19.0% vs. CABG 6.3%, RR 2.95, 95% CI 2.46–3.55, p < 0.00001)
Cui (2019) [20]	1–7.1	RCT: 5 OS:13 Total: 18	PTCA: 8550 CABG: 8982 Total:17532	All-cause mortality: Higher in PTCA arm (PTCA 10.3 vs. CABG 9.3%; HR: 1.16, 95% CI: 1.05–1.29; p = 0.005) MI: Higher in PTCA arm (PTCA 7.3% vs. CABG 4.4%; HR: 1.69, 95% CI: 1.43–2.00; p < 0.0001, I^2 = 44%) Stroke: Lower in PTCA arm (PTCA 2.6% vs. CABG 4.1%; HR: 0.67, 95% CI: 0.54–0.83; p = 0.0003, I^2 = 8%) Repeat revascularization: Higher in PTCA arm (PTCA 20.9% vs. CABG 8.6%; HR: 3.77, 95% CI: 2.76–5.16; p < 0.0001, I^2 = 78%)

MVD: Multivessel Disease; LMSD: Left Main Stem Disease; F/U: follow-up, RCT: Randomised Controlled Trials; OS: Observational Studies, MI: Myocardial Infarction, PTCA: Percutaneous Transluminal Coronary Angioplasty, CABG: Coronary Artery Bypass Grafting, HR: Hazard Ratio, Cl: Confidence Interval, RR: Relative Risk, OR: Odds Ratio

Table 2.
Meta analyses and pooled analyses of PTCA vs CABG in MVD and/or LMSD.

The first systematic review and meta-analysis that reported the outcomes of PTCA-DES vs. CABG for MVD in diabetic patients was carried out by Hakeem [16]. Of the meta-analyses identified, Huang et al. [19] included the largest number of studies; their meta-analysis consisted of a total of 19 studies (four randomised controlled trials and 15 observational studies). Moreover, it included both randomised and non-randomised studies, making it the first systematic review and meta-analyses to do so. Meanwhile, Cui's meta-analysis [20] involved three studies that compared the newer second-generation drug eluting stent (DES) Everolimus with CABG. It was also among the most recently published meta-analyses, besides having the longest period of follow-up and the highest number of diabetic patients (n = 17532).

Unlike randomised controlled trials and observational trials, meta-analyses consistently show that CABG confers a lower risk of all-cause mortality, myocardial infarction and repeat revascularization, albeit with a higher risk of stroke. We find two notable exceptions in Hakeem's [16] and Verma's [17] studies. In Hakeem's [16] study, the risk of myocardial infarction was similar in CABG and PTCA arms (10.3% versus 5.9%, RR 1.44, 95% CI 0.79 to 2.6, $p = 0.23$); however, the PTCA group displayed a trend towards higher risk of myocardial infarction. Hakeem et al. [16] attribute this phenomenon to the presence of VA CARDs trial which are responsible for the significant heterogeneity in the studies. It is noteworthy that, after excluding VA CARDs trial, MI risk attained statistical significance (RR 2.01, 95% CI 1.54 to 2.62, $p < 0.0001$) without residual heterogeneity ($I^2 = 0\%$, $p = 0.83$). Similarly, in Verma's study [17], the increase in risk of MI became significant (RR 0·57, 95% CI 0·41–0·78; $p = 0{\cdot}0004$) after VA CARDs study was excluded from the analysis ($I^2 = 0\%$).

Conversely, Huang et al. [19] excluded VA CARDS trial in their sensitivity analyses; they reported the presence of VA CARDS trial (inclusion: 8.5% DES vs. 4.6% CABG, RR 1.68, 95% CI 1.20—2.37, $p = 0.003$; exclusion: 8.6% DES vs. 4.3% CABG, RR 1.91, 95% CI 1.43–2.57, $p < 0.0001$) did not alter the overall MI rate. Nonetheless, it is to be highlighted that Huang et al. [19] analysed a total of 14 randomised and non-randomised studies. This is in sharp contrast to Hakeem et al. [16] and Verma et al. [17] who only analysed four and eight randomised studies respectively in their meta-analyses.

5. Discussion

The past decade has witnessed the increasing prevalence of diabetes, with more than a two-fold rise seen in both genders [2]. About 25–30% of patients admitted with ACS suffered from diabetes [1]. Unfortunately, compared with their non-diabetic counterparts, post-myocardial infarction complications and deaths are higher in diabetic patients after CABG or PCI [3–5]. Indeed, compared to the non-diabetic population, diabetic patients have been shown to sustain a higher composite end point of death, stroke and MI after CABG (HR: 1.55; 95% CI: 1.04 to 2.31; $p = 0.03$) or PTCA (HR: 1.53; 95% CI: 1.04 to 2.26; $p = 0.03$) in a report analysis of EXCEL trial [21]. Moreover, diabetic patients, in contrast to healthy individuals, suffered a higher rate of wound infection, neurological and renal complications, and a higher risk of stroke and readmission following CABG; this is besides the increased rates of target lesion revascularization and reinfarction after PTCA [5]. Additionally, diabetic patients are afflicted with a number of comorbidities at diagnosis, which further deteriorated their prognosis [22, 23].

Indications for revascularization therapy did not differ between diabetic and non-diabetic patients [1]. However, according to a nationwide study [4], diabetic patients tend to avoid myocardial revascularization procedures as they fear post-procedural complications and death. Furthermore, the higher frequency of proximal stenosis and extensive involvement in diabetic patients entails a higher procedural risk; this makes revascularization a less attractive treatment option for ACS [4, 24].

Nonetheless, revascularization does have some merits for diabetic patients. Several studies show that early revascularization could benefit diabetic patients by reducing the risk of adverse events [4, 25]. It was demonstrated in a meta-analysis [26] consisting of eight trials that early invasive strategy could reduce mortality rate by 36% (HR: 0.67, 95% CI: 0.45–0.99). Due to multivessel involvement and a higher risk of restenosis [5], CABG was likely the default treatment strategy for patients with diabetes in the past. Since Andreas Gruntzig introduced PTCA in 1977, notable advances have been made, which has significantly improved its success rate with a better safety profile [27]. The later introduction of drug-eluting stent (DES) drastically decreased the rate of restenosis of PTCA [27–30]. Despite these advances, whether PCI could replace CABG as an ideal treatment modality is yet to be determined.

The adverse outcomes of some treatments might not be obvious on a short-term follow-up. Additionally, the effects might alter in the long run. Long-term follow-up of patients is therefore essential. As an illustrative example, a study conducted by Pederson et al. [31] compared the cause of short-term and long-term mortality in patients treated with primary PTCA for ST segment elevation myocardial infarction. While it was shown that cardiac mortality remained the main cause of death within the first month of PTCA, the origin of death began to shift towards non-cardiac causes beyond the first month. Furthermore, Onuma et al. [8] documented that late stent and very late stent thrombosis constitute around two-thirds of stent thrombosis. To the best of our knowledge, the longest-term follow-up with regards to the outcomes of CABG and PTCA is 40 years [32]. Nonetheless, studies that follow up patients for such a long duration are few and limited. The merits of CABG significantly outweigh PTCA after four years of revascularization (pooled Absolute risk reduction = 6%), as Hakeem et al. [16] have observed. Hence, in our study, we settled on a five-year follow-up duration as the cut-off point.

When comparing the clinical outcomes of treatments of a disorder, randomised controlled trials (RCTs) are the gold standard. Yet, patients recruited in RCTs are usually specifically selected while those with multiple comorbidities are excluded; this does not reflect real-world clinical practice. Ironically, observational studies (OS) – which involve a significant level of selection, publication and treatment bias – closely mirror daily clinical practice in the hospital setting. Huang et al. [19] found that patients from observational studies enjoyed a considerably higher mortality benefit with CABG compared to their counterparts from randomised trials (Observational trials 9.6% vs. Randomised trials 11.9%, RR 0.81, 95% CI 0.71–0.92, p = 0.001). We can, therefore, infer that in the real setting, CABG is the desired choice of revascularization for patients with high risk profiles. Hence, it is essential to take into account the findings of both RCT and OS as demonstrated in our study; this allows us to determine the overall treatment effect of CABG and PTCA both clinically and statistically.

Studies — With respect to LMSD and/or MVD in diabetic patients, some notable studies are worth mentioning. The first study to demonstrate the survival advantage of CABG over PTCA among diabetic patients is the Bypass Angioplasty Revascularization Investigation (BARI) [33]. A total of 353 diabetic patients were analysed at 5-year follow up, revealing a two-fold risk of mortality rate related to PTCA. As a result, CABG was recommended as the optimal revascularization method in patients with diabetes. Though it is historically noteworthy, this study was conducted before DES and antiplatelet agents were introduced. Consequently, it has limited application to current clinical settings [5, 12, 34].

BARI study was followed by several other studies on diabetes and MVD disease that includes EAST trial, CARBI trial, RITA trial, ARTS trial, SYNTAX trial and CARDia Trial [5, 12]. We shall not discuss EAST trial, CARBI trial and RITA trial since they were too flawed for any meaningful conclusions. On the one hand, ARTS trial [35] was the first randomised trial that compared the five-year outcomes of patients with MVD treated with CABG instead of BMS. On the other hand, the first prospective randomised trial that evaluated coronary revascularization in diabetic patients was the CARDia trial [34]. Meanwhile, SYNTAX trial [15] utilised SYNTAX score to measure the extent of coronary vessels occlusion. ARTS trial, SYNTAX trial and CARDia trial consistently reported similar mortality rate coupled with excess major adverse cardiac and cerebrovascular events (MACCE) rate in the PTCA group; this called for repeat revascularization [6]. Regrettably, multiple recent studies [6, 17] have discredited these three trials as invalid on several grounds: the ARTS trial used historical control; the CARDia study was underpowered for primary composite outcome; and the SYNTAX trial involved a subgroup analysis of diabetic patients.

FREEDOM study [12] lasted from 2005 to 2010. It recruited a total of 1900 diabetic patients with MVD at 140 international centres; it was the largest prospective randomised trial. To evaluate any adverse outcomes, the patients were assigned to either CABG or PTCA with a follow-up period of between 2 to 6.75 years. This study recruited diabetic patients – high risk patients with a good distribution of SYNTAX scores coupled with optimal usage of medical therapy throughout follow-up. Consequently, it is regarded as the most outstanding trial to detect the safety and efficacy of revascularization therapies for diabetic patients with MVD. As a result, we included this study in most of the meta-analyses available. FREEDOM study is also the only study that we included in all the meta-analyses highlighted in our report. Indeed, FREEDOM Follow-On study [14] was published in 2019 with an extended median follow-up of 7.5 years to further evaluate the survival advantage of CABG over PTCA.

VA CARDS study is another study that was evaluated in numerous meta-analyses. Besides Luca's study [18], all the meta-analyses mentioned above analysed VACARDS study. VA CARDS study [16, 17, 36] aggressively searched for silent MIs that are assumed to be responsible for around one-third of the total MIs in diabetic patients. As such, following CABG, the risk of non-fatal MI was elevated drastically (CABG: 15% PCI:6.2%, HR: 3.32; 95% CI: 1.07 to 10.30). Nonetheless, we excluded this study since the follow-up duration did not meet our inclusion criteria.

BEST trial [13] compared Everolimus-eluting stent (EES) with CABG in patients with diabetes and MVD. Indeed, it represents one of the few randomised trials to do so. EES was demonstrated to be the most efficacious stent in terms of safety and efficacy thanks to its association with the lowest risk of stent thrombosis and repeat revascularization [28, 30, 37]. While evaluating how diabetic patients with MVD fared with CABG and EES for, Bangalore et al. [38] reported that EES provided comparable survival benefit to CABG (425 [10.50%] versus 414 [10.23%] events; HR = 1.12; 95% CI, 0.96–1.30; $p = 0.16$) and a lower risk of stroke (118 [2.92%] versus 157 [3.88%] events; HR = 0.76; 95% CI, 0.58–0.99; $p = 0.04$). However, this was at the expense of a higher risk of myocardial infarction (260 [6.42%] versus 166 [4.10%] events; HR = 1.64; 95% CI, 1.32–2.04; $p < 0.0001$) and repeat revascularization (889 [21.96%] versus 421 [10.40%] events; HR = 2.42; 95% CI, 2.12–2.76; $p < 0.0001$) driven by incomplete revascularization at long term. Nevertheless, it was demonstrated in BEST trial that CABG still outperformed PTCA even with EES. Due to inconsistencies in the current evidence, well-designed studies are required in the future for a more meaningful conclusion.

In LMSD, comparable adverse outcomes as well as mortality were observed in both CABG and PTCA [7, 39]. Indeed, a case could be made that the above studies were underpowered; they did not utilise Everolimus, the newer second-generation drug-eluting stent. Two of the largest randomised trials that included Everolimus are NOBEL trial [40] and EXCEL trial [41] but, unfortunately, they were not powered to study diabetic patients exclusively. A subgroup analysis of EXCEL trial [21] revealed no difference in the composite risk of all-cause mortality, stroke and myocardial infarction between CABG and PTCA in diabetic patients at 3 years (PTCA 20.7% vs. CABG 19.3%; HR: 1.03; 95% CI: 0.71 to 1.50; $p = 0.87$); however, the PTCA arm ($p = 0.01$) revealed a high risk of repeat revascularization. These results were consistent with our study findings. One exception is the higher all-cause mortality in the PTCA arm ($p = 0.046$) which included diabetic patients with high SYNTAX scores.

It should be highlighted that PCI as a substitute for CABG can only be indicated to selected LMSD patients. Patients with bifurcation lesions and unprotected LMSD yield better outcomes with CABG. Kappetein and Head [42] reported that CABG is the best treatment option for LMSD associated with bifurcation which incurs a higher risk of procedural complications, repeat revascularization and thrombosis. Yu's study [6] found similar adverse effects and mortality in both PTCA and CABG arms of unprotected LMSD patients. Nonetheless, as an unprotected left main stem occlusion is highly associated with MVD, CABG is a more reasonable revascularization modality in this patient population [42].

For MVD, in terms of adverse outcomes and mortality, a large variation has been observed in the individual studies compared to the pooled analyses or meta-analyses. This phenomenon is alluded to various study designs, types of stents or grafting and inclusion and exclusion criteria. Hence, results from individual studies should be interpreted cautiously.

To summarise, long-term survival in MVD favours CABG. In their comprehensive meta-analysis of 14 randomised trials, Herbison and Wong [43] concluded that despite significant improvement of CABG and PTCA over the past 30 years, CABG, regardless of the types of stents used, still constantly outperformed PTCA by 30% difference in survival benefit particularly in diabetic patients. In another pooled analysis [44] of 10 randomised trials involving CABG and PTCA for diabetic patients with MVD, a significantly lower five-year mortality rate was observed in the CABG arm (12.3% versus 20.0%, HR 0.70, 95% CI 0.56 to 0.87, $p = 0.014$).

Regarding adverse outcomes at long-term, it can be concluded from the above studies that, overall, CABG confer more benefits than PCI thanks to its ability to achieve complete revascularization and its lower rate of restenosis [45]. In Contini's study [9], 85.6% of CABG as compared to only 51.3% of PTCA patients could undergo complete revascularization. Similarly, Farooq et al. [46] reported that in their study, angiographic complete revascularization was only achieved in 52.8% of PTCA as opposed to 66.9% of CABG patients. Worse, the presence of diabetes further complicates the burden of incomplete revascularization. Verma and Aronson et al. [17, 21] found that diabetic population tends to present with more progressive and diffuse coronary disease. In addition, they discovered that new lesions can also form easily in the revascularization sites as diabetes progresses.

Insofar as restenosis rate is concerned, target vessel revascularization remains an unwanted effect of PCI. Multivessel angioplasty carries a higher risk of restenosis at multiple independent sites while potentially worsening the overall treatment outcomes [5]. To complicate matters, the incidence of stent thrombosis is elevated significantly with the presence of diabetes and coronary artery disease, which markedly decreases the benefit of PCI in diabetic patients [11, 21]. Although it is a more invasive procedure [18], Aronson et al. [21] noted that CABG necessitates less reintervention among both diabetic and MVD patients.

Despite its benefits, CABG carries a higher risk of stroke since antiplatelet agents are rarely used after CABG, and CABG itself is usually performed on-pump [20]. Noteworthy, in FREEDOM, 30 days after revascularization, aspirin was used 99.1% in PTCA versus 88.4% in CABG while thienopyridine was used only 98.4% and 24.6% for PTCA and CABG respectively [12, 17]. Abnormal platelets coupled with an enhanced platelet activity were observed in diabetic patients; this phenomenon leads to enhanced adhesion, activation and aggregation [47, 48]. Antiplatelet agents could therefore play a vital role in reducing the risk of thrombosis in the diabetic population. This theory is not baseless; a previous study suggested that for diabetes population afflicted with coronary artery disease, twice-daily aspirin regimen in lieu of once daily regimen could be more efficacious in hindering platelet production and platelet aggregation [49]. Given the lower frequency of antiplatelet use post CABG, a higher risk of stroke is therefore to be expected.

The utilisation of aortic manipulation in on-pump CABG is also associated with a higher risk of stroke. Aortic manipulation, it is postulated, causes atherosclerotic debris to occlude the blood vessels in the brain, with stroke as the end result. Moreover, prophylactic anti-platelet therapy might reduce the risk of stroke if provided weeks before CABG with aortic manipulation and on-pump CABG. Nonetheless, whether off-pump CABG could decrease the incidence of stroke remains debatable. On the one hand, a lower occurrence of stroke with off-pump CABG than on-pump CABG (adjusted odds ratio: 0.76, 95% CI 0.59 to 0.98, $p < 0.001$) was observed in a retrospective analysis [50] of 30,426 patients undergoing CABG surgery in 2006 and 2007. On the other hand, comparable incidence of stroke with on-pump and off-pump CABG at 5-year follow-up (OR: 0.78; 95% CI: 0.56 to 1.10; $p = 0.16$; 2.2% vs. 2.8%) [51] was reported in a recent meta-analysis of 8145 patients in six studies. After evaluating the adverse outcomes of sirolimus eluting stent versus off-pump CABG in a non-randomised trial of 207 diabetic patients with MVD, Yamagata et al. [52] observed a significantly higher rate of cerebrovascular events following off-pump CABG ($p = 0.035$) at 3 years. Based on this finding, it can be inferred that although the risk of stroke may decline with off-pump CABG, there was no significant change in the outcomes when compared with PTCA, if other factors remain unchanged. This hypothesis can only be validated by future well-designed studies.

Effect of SYNTAX score – SYNTAX score grades the complexity of coronary vessels in patients with CAD in order to determine the feasibility of CABG or PTCA [53]. Diabetes can increase the complexity of coronary lesions [54]. SYNTAX trial [15] revealed that revascularization benefits did not differ in patients with low-intermediate SYNTAX score. Conversely, among patients with intermediate-high SYNTAX score, the PTCA cohort with increasing SYNTAX score displayed increasing adverse events. Interestingly, this effect was more prominent in diabetic compared to non-diabetic individuals. We can therefore conclude that in diabetic patients, when the SYNTAX score is low, PCI can be recommended; however, when the SYNTAX score is high, CABG should be the default revascularization modality [1, 55]. This rule of thumb applies to both LMSD occlusion and MVD. Indeed, at high SYNTAX scores, a significant mortality difference was observed between CABG and PTCA in a subgroup analysis of EXCEL Trial [21] involving 554 diabetes patients. Although the EXCEL trial was underpowered for assessing mortality in diabetic patients, the trend towards improved survival could not be overlooked. Accordingly, in clinical decision making for patients with LMSD and MVD [1], the use of SYNTAX score is considered paramount. On a side note, VA CARDs trial [3] did not identify the effect of SYNTAX score on the revascularization outcomes. Admittedly, that study was underpowered with a limited number of participants and follow-up duration.

Confounding factors – We need to consider several factors when determining the long-term adverse outcomes of CABG and PCI. Glycaemic control plays a pivotal role in altering the treatment outcomes of revascularization therapy. Of all parameters, the HbA1c value is of the utmost importance [56, 57]. Interestingly, HbA1c level has been found to be associated with spontaneous platelet aggregation, reflecting underlying hypercoagulable status in diabetes [58]. Harskamp and Park [59] noted that in a study conducted by Corpus et al. [60], when the HbA1c was above 7, the rate of target vessel revascularization after PTCA was enhanced significantly (34% vs. 15%, $p = 0.02$). Moreover, a meta-analysis [61]of 16 studies also suggested that in diabetic patients receiving PTCA with a risk ratio of 1.18 (95% CI 1.10–1.27, $p = 0.016$; $I^2 = 45.8\%$), high HbA1c at baseline can independently increase the risk of major adverse cardiovascular and cerebrovascular events (MACCE). Similarly, it was revealed in an observational study [53] that the incidence of MACCE was significantly lower when HbA1c is below 7 (27.5% versus 37.4%; HR, 0.71; 95% CI, 0.52–0.97; $p = 0.03$) which is accompanied by significant reduction of repeat revascularization (19.9% versus 29.5%; HR, 0.66; 95% CI, 0.47–0.93; $p = 0.02$). It was found that this benefit was maximised when the residual SYNTAX score was above four.

Interestingly, potential determinants of mortality of PCI include psychological factors as well. A recent study [62] with a 12-year follow-up revealed that patients with higher feelings of being disabled one month after PCI had a significantly higher mortality rate (43.5% vs. 23.1%; HR = 2.53, 95% CI = 1.30–4.90, $p = 0.001$). Due to the paucity of reliable data, future robust studies are required to determine the relationship between psychological states and PCI mortality.

It is known that diabetes can lead to a thrombotic state via various mechanisms [63]. Antiplatelet agents are crucial in minimising the risks of hypercoagulability. For several decades, aspirin and clopidogrel have been used as the standard antiplatelet regimens. However, newer antiplatelet agents (such as Ticagrelor and Prasugrel) appear to generate more favourable outcomes than the older medications, especially in diabetic patients [64, 65]. A meta-analysis [66] of seven randomised controlled trials involving 58,591 patients with ACS revealed that patients with Ticagrelor or Prasugrel had a significant decline in mortality (2.9% vs. 3.4%, OR = 0.87, 95% CI 0.79–0.95, $p = 0.002$), recurrent myocardial infarction (4.2% vs. 5.2%, OR = 0.80, 95% CI 0.74–0.87, $p < 0.0001$) and definite in-stent thrombosis (0.9% vs. 1.7%, OR = 0.52, 95% CI 0.43–0.63, $p < 0.0001$) without an elevation of major bleeding complications (5% vs. 4.7%, OR = 1.06 95% CI 0.96–1.17, $p = 0.25$). These findings corroborate the OPTIMUS trial [59] that demonstrated a greater inhibition of platelet activity by Prasugrel than Clopidogrel (89.3 vs. 27.7%, $p = 0.0001$). Nonetheless, the clinical efficacy and safety of Ticagrelor and Prasugrel post revascularization therapy is yet to be proven to date. Hence, well-designed studies looking at this aspect are warranted.

6. Limitations

Despite our best effort to include similar studies and exclude studies which present significant heterogeneity from other studies, a number of variables still exist between the studies as a result of various inclusion and exclusion criteria and study designs. We also admit that definition of adverse outcomes, follow-up duration and types of grafting which differ from one study to another can potentially affect the treatment outcomes. In addition, the aforementioned studies did not capture factors such as HbA1c level, SYNTAX score, treatment of diabetes and psychological factors. Moreover, only a limited number of studies were analysed since we excluded studies that are not published in English. Furthermore, since only a limited number of studies utilised EES, the results should be interpreted with caution when applied to the clinical setting where EES is widely performed. Robust studies utilising EES are warranted in the future. Lastly, several observational studies were recruited in our study where they posed inherent bias; nonetheless, it is unlikely that the results would differ considerably after exclusion of the observational trials.

7. Future directions

The coronary vessels of diabetic patients are lined with the more extensive and severe atherosclerotic plaque. This has given rise to hybrid coronary revascularization (HCR) [67]. HCR combines the essence of CABG and PCI to mitigate issues related to MVD [68]. In HCR, CABG is performed in the left anterior descending artery while PCI is utilised to open up the other occluded vessels [69, 70]. A robotic procedure is used for this minimally invasive CABG procedure where only small incisions rather than a midline incision are required. In this best-of-both-worlds strategy, a minimally-invasive off-pump left internal mammary graft is connected to the blocked left anterior descending artery, and a stent is then placed from the left main to the left circumflex artery.

HCR is safer and more effective than CABG or PCI. By avoiding sternotomy, cardiopulmonary bypass and most importantly, aortic manipulation, HCR is associated with a lower infection, transfusion and prolonged recovery rate and risk of stroke [62, 64, 71, 72]. Since diabetic patients are prone to more frequent infections with a slower healing rate, HCR would benefit them enormously.

HCR had a similar all-cause mortality (6.4% for HCR vs.9.2% for CABG; $p = 0.69$), myocardial infarction (4.3% vs. 7.2%; $p = 0.30$) and repeat revascularization (37.2% vs. 45.4%; $p = 0.38$), stroke (2.1% vs. 4.1%; $p = 0.35$) and MACCE s (45.2% vs. 53.4%; $p = 0.39$) in a randomised study [62] of 191 patients with MVD at five years. However, a trend towards better outcomes favours HCR instead of the conventional CABG. In a prospective study [61] at Fuwai Hospital in Japan, 120 diabetic patients were enrolled in the HCR arm and 240 patients in the off-pump CABG arm. A follow-up of MACCE events after three years reported a lower rate of stroke in the CABG arm (0% vs. 3.6% at 3 years; $p = 0.046$).

We anticipate that HCR will be widely used in the near future [73]. Currently, there is insufficient evidence to guide the application of the procedures to diabetic patients [66, 67, 74]. Hence, future robust studies on long-term follow up are needed.

8. Conclusion

As an option in diabetic patients, revascularization is dictated by the complexity and nature of the coronary vessels involved. A low SYNTAX score favours PCI as an alternative to CABG. However, CABG is recommended at an intermediate-high SYNTAX score. Meanwhile, in multivessel involvement or complex CAD, CABG remains the mainstay of treatment. In left main stem occlusion, when the disease is accompanied by bifurcation or is classified as unprotected left main stem disease, CABG could offer better treatment outcomes. Factors such as patient's quality of life and cost effectiveness of therapy, coupled with other clinical factors and short-term clinical outcomes, should not be ignored in clinical decision making; these should be communicated clearly and effectively to patients in order to have their informed consent. The implementation of shared decision making is vital when formulating the best revascularization option; patients' preferences, values and needs are to be respected and honoured.

Acknowledgements

The author would like to express his gratitude to Cheang Jia Min, Jeffrey Cheah School of Medicine & Health Sciences, Monash University Malaysia for research assistance, and Nageeb Gounjaria, Center for Bioethics and Medical Humanities, Universitas Gadjah Mada, Indonesia for proofreading and editing the manuscript.

Author details

Ahmad Farouk Musa[1,2]

1 Jeffrey Cheah School of Medicine and Health Sciences, Monash University Malaysia, Selangor Darul Ehsan, Malaysia

2 Victorian Heart Institute, Monash University, Melbourne, Australia

*Address all correspondence to: farouk@monash.edu

References

[1] Neumann F-J, Sousa-Uva M, Ahlsson A, et al. 2018 ESC/EACTS guidelines on myocardial revascularization. European Heart Journal. 2019;**40**(2):87-165

[2] Zhou B, Lu Y, Hajifathalian K, Bentham J, et al. Worldwide trends in diabetes since 1980: A pooled analysis of 751 population-based studies with 4· 4 million participants. The Lancet. 2016;**387**(10027):1513-1530

[3] King SB, Marshall JJ, Tummala PE. Revascularization for coronary artery disease: Stents versus bypass surgery. Annual Review of Medicine. 2010;**61**(1):199-213

[4] Gustafsson I, Hvelplund A, Hansen KW, et al. Underuse of an invasive strategy for patients with diabetes with acute coronary syndrome: A nationwide study. Open Heart. 2015;(1):e000165

[5] Singh M, Arora R, Kodumuri V, Khosla S, Jawad E. Coronary revascularization in diabetic patients: Current state of evidence. Experimental & Clinical Cardiology. 2011;**16**(1):16-22

[6] Yu X, He J, Luo Y, et al. Influence of diabetes mellitus on long-term outcomes of patients with unprotected left main coronary artery disease treated with either drug-eluting stents or coronary artery bypass grafting. International Heart Journal. 2015;**56**(1):43-48

[7] Lee K, Ahn JM, Yoon Y-H, et al. Long-yerm (10-Year) outcomes of stenting or bypass surgery for left main coronary artery disease in patients with and without diabetes mellitus. Journal of the American Heart Association. 2020;**9**(8):e015372

[8] Onuma Y, Wykrzykowska JJ, Garg S, Vranckx P, Serruys PW. 5-year follow-up of coronary revascularization in diabetic patients with multivessel coronary artery disease. JACC: Cardiovascular Interventions. 2011;**4**(3):317-323

[9] Contini GA, Nicolini F, Fortuna D, et al. Five-year outcomes of surgical or percutaneous myocardial revascularization in diabetic patients. International Journal of Cardiology. 2013;**168**(2):1028-1033

[10] Kim YG, Park DW, Lee WS, et al. Influence of diabetes mellitus on long-term (five-year) outcomes of drug-eluting stents and coronary artery bypass grafting for multivessel coronary revascularization. The American Journal of Cardiology. 2012;**109**(11):1548-1557

[11] Moshkovitz Y, Mohr R, Medalion B, Hyam E, Herz I, Deitch I, et al. Drug-eluting stents compared with bilateral internal thoracic artery grafts for diabetic patients. The Annals of Thoracic Surgery. 2012;**94**(5):1455-1462

[12] Farkouh ME, Domanski M, Sleeper LA, et al. Strategies for multivessel revascularization in patients with diabetes. The New England Journal of Medicine. 2012;**367**(25):2375

[13] Park SJ, Ahn JM, Kim YH, et al. Trial of everolimus-eluting stents or bypass surgery for coronary disease. New England Journal of Medicine. 2015;**372**(13):1204-1212

[14] Farkouh ME, Domanski M, Dangas GD, et al. Long-term survival following multivessel revascularization in patients with diabetes. Journal of the American College of Cardiology. 2019;**73**(6):629-638

[15] Kappetein AP, Head SJ, Morice M-C, et al. Treatment of complex coronary artery disease in patients with diabetes: 5-year results comparing outcomes of bypass surgery and percutaneous coronary intervention in the SYNTAX trial †. European Journal of Cardio-Thoracic Surgery. 2013;**43**(5):1006-1013

[16] Hakeem A, Garg N, Bhatti S, Rajpurohit N, Ahmed Z, Uretsky BF. Effectiveness of percutaneous coronary intervention with drug-eluting stents compared with bypass surgery in diabetics with multivessel coronary disease: Comprehensive systematic review and meta-analysis of randomised clinical data. Journal of the American Heart Association. 2013;**2**(4):e000354

[17] Verma S, Farkouh ME, Yanagawa B, et al. Comparison of coronary artery bypass surgery and percutaneous coronary intervention in patients with diabetes: A meta-analysis of randomised controlled trials. The Lancet Diabetes & Endocrinology. 2013;**1**(4):317-328

[18] De Luca G, Schaffer A, Verdoia M, Suryapranata H. Meta-analysis of 14 trials comparing bypass grafting vs. drug-eluting stents in diabetic patients with multivessel coronary artery disease. Nutrition, Metabolism and Cardiovascular Diseases. 2014;**24**(4):344-354

[19] Huang F, Lai W, Chan C, et al. Comparison of bypass surgery and drug-eluting stenting in diabetic patients with left main and/or multivessel disease: A systematic review and meta-analysis of randomised and nonrandomized studies. Cardiology Journal. 2015;**22**(2):123-134

[20] Cui K, Lyu S, Song X, et al. Drug-eluting stent versus coronary artery bypass grafting for diabetic patients with multivessel and/or left main coronary artery disease: A meta-analysis. Angiology. 2019;**70**(8):765-773

[21] Milojevic M, Serruys PW, Sabik JF, et al. Bypass surgery or stenting for left main coronary artery disease in patients with diabetes. Journal of the American College of Cardiology. 2019;**73**(13):1616-1628

[22] Foussas SG. Acute coronary syndromes and diabetes mellitus. Hellenic Journal of Cardiology. 2016;**57**(5):375-377

[23] Giraldez RR, Clare RM, Lopes RD, et al. Prevalence and clinical outcomes of undiagnosed diabetes mellitus and prediabetes among patients with high-risk non–ST-segment elevation acute coronary syndrome. American Heart Journal. 2013;**165**(6):918-925

[24] Zand Parsa AF, Ziai H, Haghighi L. The impact of cardiovascular risk factors on the site and extent of coronary artery disease. Cardiovascular Journal of Africa. 2012;**23**(4):197-199

[25] O'Donoghue ML, Vaidya A, Afsal R, et al. An invasive or conservative strategy in patients with diabetes mellitus and non–ST-segment elevation acute coronary syndromes. Journal of the American College of Cardiology. 2012;**60**(2):106-111

[26] Jobs A, Mehta SR, Montalescot G, et al. Optimal timing of an invasive strategy in patients with non-ST-elevation acute coronary syndrome: A meta-analysis of randomised trials. The Lancet. 2017;**390**(10096):737-746

[27] Sheth SD, Giugliano RP. Coronary artery stents: Advances in technology. Hospital Practice. 2014;**42**(4):83-91

[28] Iqbal J, Gunn J, Serruys PW. Coronary stents: Historical development, current status and future directions. British Medical Bulletin. 2013;**106**(1):193-211

[29] Alfonso C, Cohen M. Transradial artery catheterization in the United States. Cardiac Interventions Today. 2014:29-34

[30] Katz G, Harchandani B, Shah B. Drug-eluting stents: The past, present, and future. Current Atherosclerosis Reports. 2015;**17**(3):11

[31] Pedersen F, Butrymovich V, Kelbæk H, et al. Short-and long-term cause of death in patients treated with primary PCI for STEMI. Journal of the American College of Cardiology. 2014;**64**(20):2101-2108

[32] Milojevic M, Thuijs DJ, Head SJ, et al. Life-long clinical outcome after the first myocardial revascularization procedures: 40-year follow-up after coronary artery bypass grafting and percutaneous coronary intervention in Rotterdam. Interactive Cardiovascular and Thoracic surgery. 2019;**28**(6):852-859

[33] Alderman E, Andrews K, Bost J, Bourassa M. Comparison of coronary bypass surgery with angioplasty in patients with multivessel disease. The New England Journal of Medicine. 1996;**335**(4):217-225

[34] Kapur A, Hall RJ, Malik IS, et al. Randomised comparison of percutaneous coronary intervention with coronary artery bypass grafting in diabetic patients. Journal of the American College of Cardiology. 2010;**55**(5):432-440

[35] Serruys PW, Ong ATL, van Herwerden LA, et al. Five-year outcomes after coronary stenting versus bypass surgery for the treatment of multivessel disease. Journal of the American College of Cardiology. 2005;**46**(4):575-581

[36] Kamalesh M, Sharp TG, Tang XC, et al. Percutaneous coronary intervention versus coronary bypass surgery in United States Veterans with diabetes. Journal of the American College of Cardiology. 2013;**61**(8):808-816

[37] Bangalore S, Kumar S, Fusaro M, et al. Outcomes with various drug eluting or bare metal stents in patients with diabetes mellitus: Mixed treatment comparison analysis of 22 844 patient years of follow-up from randomised trials. BMJ. 2012;**345**:e5170

[38] Bangalore LS, Guo LY, Samadashvili LZ, Blecker LS, Xu LJ, Hannan LE. Everolimus eluting stents versus coronary artery bypass graft surgery for patients with diabetes mellitus and multivessel disease. Circulation: Cardiovascular Interventions. 2015;**8**(7):e002626

[39] Park S-J, Park D-W. Diabetes in myocardial revascularization for left main coronary artery disease: Predictor or decision maker? Journal of the American College of Cardiology. 2019;**73**(13):1629-1632

[40] Holm NR, Mäkikallio T, Lindsay MM, et al. Percutaneous coronary angioplasty versus coronary artery bypass grafting in the treatment of unprotected left main stenosis: Updated 5-year outcomes from the randomised, non-inferiority NOBLE trial. The Lancet. 2020;**395**(10219):191-199

[41] Stone GW, Sabik JF, Serruys PW, et al. Everolimus-eluting stents or bypass surgery for left main coronary artery disease. New England Journal of Medicine. 2016;**375**(23):2223-2235

[42] Kappetein AP, Head S. CABG, stents, or hybrid procedures for left main disease? Eurointervention. Journal of Europcr in Collaboration with the Working Group on Interventional Cardiology of the European Society of Cardiology. 2015;**11**:V111-V114

[43] Herbison P, Wong C-K. Has the difference in mortality between percutaneous coronary intervention and coronary artery bypass grafting in people with heart disease and diabetes changed over the years? A systematic review and meta-regression. BMJ Open. 2015;**5**(12):e010055

[44] Hlatky MA, Boothroyd DB, Bravata DM, Boersma E, Booth J, Brooks MM, et al. Coronary artery bypass surgery compared with percutaneous coronary interventions for multivessel disease: A collaborative analysis of individual patient data from ten randomised trials. The Lancet. 2009;**373**(9670):1190-1197

[45] Aronson D, Edelman ER. Coronary artery disease and diabetes mellitus. Cardiology Clinics. 2014;**32**(3):439-455

[46] Farooq V, Serruys PW, Garcia-Garcia HM, et al. The negative impact of incomplete angiographic revascularization on clinical outcomes and its association with total occlusions. Journal of the American College of Cardiology. 2013;**61**(3):282-294

[47] Ferreiro JL, Angiolillo DJ. Diabetes and antiplatelet therapy in acute coronary syndrome. Circulation. 2011;**123**(7):798-813

[48] Kaur R, Kaur M, Singh J. Endothelial dysfunction and platelet hyperactivity in type 2 diabetes mellitus: Molecular insights and therapeutic strategies. Cardiovascular Diabetology. 2018;**17**(1)

[49] Capodanno D, Patel A, Dharmashankar K, et al. Pharmacodynamic effects of different aspirin dosing regimens in type 2 diabetes mellitus patients with coronary artery disease. Journal of the American College of Cardiology. 2011;**57**(14):E1910

[50] Li Z, Denton T, Yeo KK, et al. Off-pump bypass surgery and postoperative stroke: California Coronary Bypass Outcomes Reporting Program. The Annals of Thoracic Surgery. 2010;**90**(3):753-759

[51] Smart NA, Dieberg G, King N. Long-term outcomes of on- versus off-pump coronary artery bypass grafting. Journal of the American College of Cardiology. 2018;**71**(9):983-991

[52] Yamagata KI, Kataoka Y, Kokubu N, et al. A 3-year clinical outcome after percutaneous coronary intervention using sirolimus-eluting stent and off-pump coronary artery bypass grafting for the treatment of diabetic patients with multivessel disease. Circulation Journal: Official Journal of the Japanese Circulation Society. 2010;**74**(4):671-678

[53] Sianos G, Morel MA, Kappetein AP, et al. The SYNTAX Score: An angiographic tool grading the complexity of coronary artery disease. EuroIntervention. 2005;**1**(2):219-227

[54] Tanaka T, Seto S, Yamamoto K, Kondo M, Otomo T. An assessment of risk factors for the complexity of coronary artery disease using the SYNTAX score. Cardiovascular Intervention and Therapeutics. 2013;**28**(1):16-21

[55] Head SJ, Milojevic M, Daemen J, et al. Mortality after coronary artery bypass grafting versus percutaneous coronary intervention with stenting for coronary artery disease: A pooled analysis of individual patient data. The Lancet. 2018;**391**(10124):939-948

[56] Wang TKM, Woodhead A, Ramanathan T, Pemberton J. Relationship between diabetic variables and outcomes after coronary artery bypass grafting in diabetic patients. Heart, Lung and Circulation. 2017;**26**(4):371-375

[57] Musa A, Cheong XP, Yap C, Dillon J, Nordin R. Does diabetes mellitus increase the mortality risk in coronary artery disease patients undergoing coronary artery bypass grafting surgery at the National Heart Institute of Kuala Lumpur? Journal of Diabetes, Metabolic Disorders & Control. 2018;**5**:141-143

[58] Hwang KJ, Lee HS, Song BY, et al. Glycemic control status after percutaneous coronary intervention and long-term clinical outcomes in patients with type 2 diabetes mellitus. Circulation: Cardiovascular Interventions. 2017;**10**(4):e004157-e

[59] Harskamp RE, Park DW. Percutaneous coronary intervention in diabetic patients: Should choice of stents be influenced? Expert Review of Cardiovascular Therapy. 2013;**11**(5):541-553

[60] Corpus RA, George PB, House JA, et al. Optimal glycemic control is associated with a lower rate of target vessel revascularization in treated type II diabetic patients undergoing elective percutaneous coronary intervention. Journal of the American College of Cardiology. 2004;**43**(1):8-14

[61] Xu X, Wang R, Wang Y, Cai S. Glycosylated haemoglobin levels and clinical outcomes in diabetic patients receiving percutaneous coronary interventions: A meta-analysis of cohort studies. International Journal of Cardiology. 2015;**190**(1):143-147

[62] Bergmann MJ, Utens EMWJ, de Jager TAJ, et al. Feelings of being disabled as a prognostic factor for mortality in men and women post-PCI up to 12 years. International Journal of Cardiology. 2017;**249**:107-111

[63] Pomero F, Minno M, Fenoglio L, et al. Is diabetes a hypercoagulable state? A critical appraisal. Acta Diabetologica. 2015;**52**(6):1007-1016

[64] Alexopoulos D, Xanthopoulou I, Mavronasiou E, et al. Randomised assessment of ticagrelor versus prasugrel antiplatelet effects in patients with diabetes. Diabetes Care. 2013;**36**(8):2211-2216

[65] Angiolillo DJ, Badimon JJ, Saucedo JF, et al. A pharmacodynamic comparison of prasugrel vs. high-dose clopidogrel in patients with type 2 diabetes mellitus and coronary artery disease: Results of the Optimising anti-Platelet Therapy In diabetes MellitUS (OPTIMUS)-3 Trial. European Heart Journal. 2011;**32**(7):838-846

[66] Navarese EP, Verdoia M, Schaffer A, et al. Ischaemic and bleeding complications with new, compared to standard, ADP-antagonist regimens in acute coronary syndromes: A meta-analysis of randomised trials. QJM: An International Journal of Medicine. 2011;**104**(7):561-569

[67] Song Z, Shen L, Zheng Z, et al. One-stop hybrid coronary revascularization versus off-pump coronary artery bypass in patients with diabetes mellitus. The Journal of Thoracic and Cardiovascular Surgery. 2016;**151**(6):1695-1701

[68] Tajstra M, Hrapkowicz T, Hawranek M, et al. Hybrid coronary revascularization in selected patients with multivessel disease. JACC: Cardiovascular Interventions. 2018;**11**(9):847-852

[69] Hage A, Giambruno V, Jones P, et al. Hybrid coronary revascularization versus off-pump coronary artery bypass grafting: Comparative effectiveness analysis with long-term follow-up. Journal of the American Heart Association. 2019;**8**(24):e014204

[70] Kayatta MO, Halkos ME, Puskas JD. Hybrid coronary revascularization for the treatment of multivessel coronary artery disease. Annals of Cardiothoracic Surgery. 2018;**7**(4):500-505

[71] Harskamp RE, Brennan JM, Xian Y, et al. Practice patterns and clinical outcomes after hybrid coronary revascularization in the United States: An analysis from the society of thoracic surgeons adult cardiac database. Circulation. 2014;**130**(11):872-879

[72] Harskamp RE, Walker PF, Alexander JH, et al. Clinical outcomes of hybrid coronary revascularization versus coronary artery bypass surgery in patients with diabetes mellitus. American Heart Journal. 2014;**168**(4):471-478

[73] Saha T, Naqvi SY, Goldberg S. Hybrid revascularization: A review. Cardiology. 2018;**140**(1):35-44

[74] Repossini A, Tespili M, Saino A, et al. Hybrid coronary revascularization in 100 patients with multivessel coronary disease. The Annals of Thoracic Surgery. 2014;**98**(2):574-581

Chapter 8

Left Main Coronary Artery Disease: Current Updates on CABG versus PCI

Sridhar Kasturi

Abstract

Most patients of LMCA disease are symptomatic and at high risk of cardiovascular (CV) events, since occlusion compromises flow, and it is associated with >20% mortality at 1 year. Coronary artery by-pass graft (CABG) is the main mode of revascularization procedure for significant left-main coronary artery (LMCA) disease unless contraindicated or unsuitable for surgery, and in patients with complex coronary anatomy. Percutaneous coronary intervention (PCI) of left-main (LM) is emerging as an alternative to CABG especially in patients with low syntax score with suitable coronary anatomy for PCI, and life-saving emergency situations like acute coronary syndrome (ACS) with hemodynamically unstable, and high risk group patients who are unsuitable coronary anatomy for grafting or due to associated co-morbidities.

Keywords: CABG, PCI, LMCA, clinical trails, syntax score, current updates

1. Introduction

LMCA arises from the left coronary sinus in majority of patients, most often divides into two major branches; 1) Left anterior descending (LAD) is the larger vessel in majority of patients, supplies anterior aspect of left ventricle and anterior portion of septum. 2) left circumflex (LCX) supplies left lateral and posterior aspect of left ventricle (LV). In some patients, it trifurcates into LAD, LCX and Ramus branches, and in 1% of the population, may present like atretic segment or both branches may arise directly from the aorta via separate ostia [1]. LMCA has an average length of 10.8 ± 5.2 mm (range 2–23 mm), an average diameter of 4.9 ± 0.8, and supplies more than 75% of the blood supply to the LV in a right dominant system and almost 100% supply to the LV in a left dominant system [2].

LM has higher elastic component that may lead to stent under expansion & recoiling which necessitates use of stents with sufficient radial strength. LM disease more often associated with hard fibro- calcific plaques with tapering of the vessel [3]. Conventionally, an angiographic cut off of >50% diameter stenosis (equivalent to >75% area stenosis) has been used to indicate hemodynamic significance, as suggested

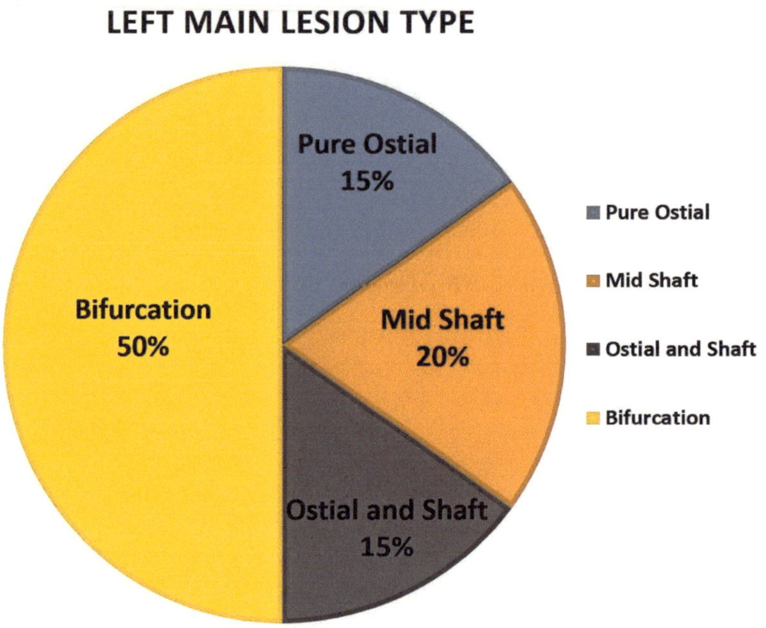

Figure 1.
Type of lesions involving left main.

by early work in an animal model by Gould that demonstrated a reduction in hyperaemic flow. Significant LMCA disease defined as >50% narrowing is found in 4 to 6% of patients who undergo coronary angiography, and it involves ostium in 15%, mid segment in 20%, ostium to Proximal shaft in 15%, and LM bifurcation lesions in 50% of patients. **Figure 1** across lesions beyond 50% degree of stenosis of LM [4].

Clinical Presentation: LM disease most often presents with ACS in >63%, and stable ischemic heart disease in 37% of cases, and sometimes with life threatening arrhythmias and sudden death. Ostial stenosis is more often seen in women (44 vs. 20%) compared to men [5]. Oveido et al. demonstrated that LM lesion extending into the proximal LAD, LCX or both may be seen in 90%, 60.4% and 62% of patients, respectively, whereas isolated ostia of LAD & LCx lesions without extending to LM were seen in 9.3% and 17.1% of patients, respectively [6].

1.1 Etiology

Atherosclerosis is the most common cause of LMCA disease, and other causes of LMCA disease are rare. Diseases involving ascending aorta may also cause LMCA obstruction such as aortic dissection, aortic aneurysm, Takayasu arteritis, systemic vascular disorders, thromboembolism to LM, and sometimes it might be due to iatrogenic causes like trans-catheter valve implants in a lower coronary origin or shallow sinuses of Valsalva, and iatrogenic catheter induced traumatic dissection or spasm of LM [1].

2. Replace this text with your section heading

2.1 Non-invasive predictors of LMCA disease

Myocardial perfusion scan indicative of significant LM disease is presence of multiple large perfusion defects in the LAD and LCX territories mainly associated with exercise induced transient ischemic dilation (TID) of left ventricle, and increased lung uptake of tracer. Probability of LM disease more likely in the presence of stress-induced sustained ventricular tachyarrhythmia or non-sustained ventricular tachyarrhythmia >30 seconds or ST-segment elevation, exercise LV ejection fraction ≤35%, and appearance of new regional wall motion abnormality (RWMA) involving >2 segments at a low-dose dobutamine stress test (≤10 mg/kg per minute), inducible ischemia at a low heart rate (<120 beats per minute) or at low level of exercise test, and exercise induced fall in systolic BP [7].

2.2 Assessment of LM with Computed Tomography (CT) and Magnetic Resonance Imaging (MRI)

Multi-slice spiral computed tomography (MSCT) is accurate in identifying LM lesions with >50% narrowing with a sensitivity of 97% and specificity of 86% compared with angiography, and CMRI detection of coronary lesions in heavily calcified coronary segments is more reliable than by cardiac CT. Overall, the accuracy of MSCT for detection of angiographic in-stent restenosis (ISR) of LM was 93% with 100% sensitivity, 91% specificity, and 100% negative predictive values [8]. The DISCOVER FLOW trial demonstrated that Fractional flow reserve (FFR) CT could dramatically improve the diagnostic accuracy of CT imaging without the need for invasive FFR imaging [9].

2.3 Angiographic assessment of LMCA

Coronary angiography remains the gold standard diagnostic technique for the diagnosis of clinically important LMCA disease. Angiography is poor in assessing characterization of tissue or plaque (except for calcium, aneurysms, coarse ulcerations, or large dissections) and features associated with suboptimal stent deployment. In order to avoid precipitating myocardial ischemia in patients with severe LMCA disease perform angiography with careful manipulations of catheters, limited angiographic images with minimal contrast dose to avoid procedure related sudden events. Sometimes, Ostial LMCA stenosis is very difficult to make out on angiography and it should be suspected if there is any pressure damp and absence of reflex of dye in to the coronary sinus. Disease involving entire LMCA may be underestimated due to lack of reference segment, and in such cases indirect assessment of LMCA diameter and size can be estimated by using Finet's and Murray's law using main branch (MB) and side branch (SB) diameters [10, 11]. Angio is also poor at assessing lesion calcification due to its low sensitivity in detecting calcium (45–50%), and this may lead to underestimation of calcium contributing to procedure delay, failure of PCI due to absence of plaque modification resulting in under expansion, dissection, failure to cross lesions with balloons and stents, and dislodgement of stents. Intravascular ultrasound (IVUS) and Optical coherence tomography (OCT) have better sensitivity 80% vs. 50% in detecting calcium compared to angiography.

2.4 Usefulness of IVI and Functional testing to assess LM disease

Angiographic assessment of borderline LM lesions (30–70%) is inaccurate with significant inter-observer variability whereas the reproducibility and accuracy of the angiographic evaluation of LM lesions <30% and ≥ 70% is excellent Thus, revascularization strategies of borderline lesions based solely on the angiography may lead to incorrect revascularization strategies due to improper assessment of LMCA severity which might adversely affects clinical outcomes because of low graft patency rates and up to a 6-fold higher rate of atherosclerotic disease progression of bypassed native coronary vessels [12]. Intravascular imaging is helpful in assessing severity and to decide revascularization strategies particularly in patients with angiography showing doubtful, inaccurate, ambiguous lesions, intermediate lesions without any noninvasive evaluation of inducible ischemia or and whenever no correlation between angiography lesion severity and clinical symptoms. OCT is not considered as ideal imaging option for ostio-proximal LM lesions and might be limited in case of large vessel (>5.5 mm diameter) but the technique superior to IVUS in identification of thrombus, stent under expansion, struts mal apposition and edge dissection thrombus, due to its better spatial resolution. Lesions involving mid and distal LM can be adequately visualized by OCT imaging modality with high resolution images and comparable results with IVUS. OCT can reveal more detail, whereas IVUS provides more insight in deeper layers of the coronary arteries. The expert consensus group stated that IVUS and OCT are equivalent and both superior to coronary angiogram (CAG) guidance [13]. However, an extensive Random clinical trial (RCT) that addresses superiority of OCT guidance is currently still lacking.

Based on the findings of LITRO study, patients with intermediate LM stenosis between 25% and 60% lesions with minimal luminal area (MLA) of ≥6 mm^2 revascularization of LM (**Figure 2**) can be safely deferred with favorable outcomes at 2 years

Proposed published cut-off for LMCA MLA

Study	Methods	Cut-off MLA (mm^2)
Jasti et al, 2004	IVUS vs FFR <0.75, n=55	5.9
Fassa et al, 2005	Population based normal range, n=214	7.5
De la Torre Hernandez et al, 2011	Prospective clinical validation, n=354	6
Park et al, 2014	IVUS vs FFR <0.8, n=112	4.5

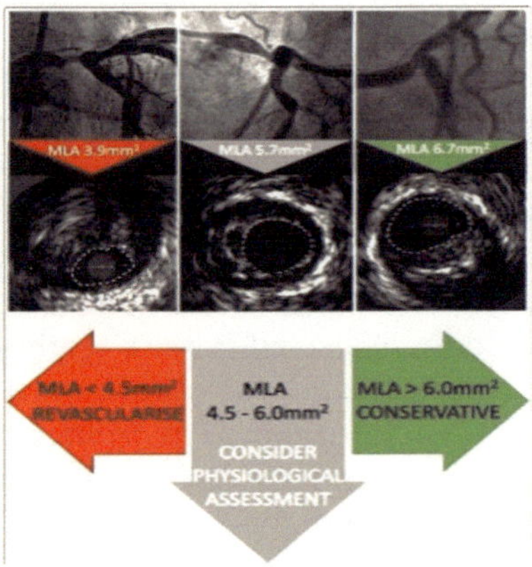

MLA measured by OCT is significantly smaller than by IVUS (FD-OCT MLA being 10-15% lower than IVUS MLA

Figure 2.
Mean luminal area of LMCA by IVUS from various studies.

of follow-up (cardiac death-free survival of 97.7%). Nearly 30% of patients with mild disease of LMCA with less than 30% narrowing had an MLA of <6 mm^2, whereas 43% of patients with angiographic LM stenosis ≥50% had a prognostically favorable MLA of ≥6 mm^2 [14].

S J Park group suggested the MLA cut-off for FFR < 0.80 was 4.5 mm^2 for south Asians with a sensitivity of 77% and a negative predictive value of 75% [15]. Based on results of DEFINE-FLAIR and iFR-SWEDEHEART studies cut off value of instantaneous wave free ratio (iFR) for deferring revascularization of lesions is >0.89. However, if the FFR is between 0.81 and 0.85, then the hemodynamic significance of the LM lesion cannot be accurately determined if the combined FFR of the LM and the downstream disease is ≤0.45. In such situations, IVUS or OCT imaging assessment of mean luminal areas will be helpful to decide whether revascularization is required or not, IVUS MLA < 4.5MM^2 needs revascularization, and IVUS MLA is between 4.5mm^2 and 6mm^2 requires FFR assessment after treating downstream vessel to decide revascularization of LM is required or not based on FFR value. > 0.80 or < 0.80, and revascularization should be avoided if IVUS measured LM MLA > 6 mm^2 [16].

2.5 Early experience of PCI

Most patients of LMCA disease are symptomatic and at high risk of CV events, since occlusion compromises flow to at least 75% of the LV, and it is associated >20% mortality at 1 year. Presently four management strategies recommended for LMCA disease: medical therapy, PCI, or surgical revascularization (CABG) either off pump or on-pump, and hybrid (CABG + PCI) procedures. For all practical purposes, CABG is the main mode of revascularization procedure for significant LMCA disease unless contraindicated or unsuitable for surgery due to better long term results particularly in diabetics, and in patients with complex coronary anatomy, and it was based on superior results observed in 3 randomized trials conducted in 70's and 80's - VA study [17], ECSS study [18], and CASS study [19]. CABG improved survival and symptoms mainly in patients with triple Vessel Disease and LMCA disease associated with severe LV dysfunction, and positive exercise induced ischemia. 150 patients of Left Main Disease in VA and EU RCT study showed 5 years Mortality was 36.5% v/s 16% in Medical treated v/s CABG group. CASS registry consisting of 1484 patients showed significantly improved survival rate at the end of 10 years and 15 years follow up in CABG treated patients v/s Medically treated patients [20]. Until recently CABG was the only option considered for significant LMCA disease and PCI was regarded as a harmful procedure with poor acute and long term results. However, PCI of LM is emerging as an alternative to CABG especially in patients with low syntax score with suitable coronary anatomy for PCI, and life-saving emergency situations like ACS with hemodynamically unstable, and high risk group patients who are unsuitable coronary anatomy for grafting or due to associated co-morbidities.

Andreas Gruntzig was the 1st person to perform first plain balloon angioplasty of LMCA in 1976. Later, O'Keefe et al. reported 127 angioplasty procedures of LMCA lesions with a procedural mortality of 9.1% and 3-year survival rate of 36% [21]. The beginning era of LM interventional management with plain balloon angioplasty was associated with a high mortality and morbidity due to abrupt vessel closure and acute stent thrombosis. Subsequently, Era of Bare-metal stents showed high restenosis and repeat revascularization rates with an increased incidence of sudden cardiac deaths.

In 1994 a meta-analysis of 7 studies that randomized a total of 2649 patients to medical therapy or CABG, showed survival advantage of surgery over medical therapy for patients with LMCA or three-vessel disease [22]. Later S J Park reported series of 42 patients with stenting of LMCA with immediate and late outcomes in 1998 and suggested stenting of unprotected LMCA as a safe and effective alternative to CABG in a carefully selected patient with normal LV Function with a 22% restenosis at 6 months follow up [23]. Erglis et al. analyzed results of PCI with stenting of LM, 103 patients with stable angina treated with either paclitaxel-eluting stent or bare-metal stent, IVUS and CB were used prior to stenting, which resulted in binary restenosis in 11 (22%) bare-metal stent and in 3 (6%) paclitaxel-eluting stent patients ($p = 0.021$) [24]. ISAR-LM randomized trial, comparing sirolimus-eluting stent vs. Paclitaxel-eluting stent, revealed no significant differences were reported in the composite outcome of death, MI, and TLR at 1 year follow-up, and no difference seen in TLF and 2-year LM-specific revascularization [25].

2.6 Early experience of PCI of LMCA with 1st generation DES

Acute and long term out comes of PCI of LMCA compared with CABG studied in 4 major trials (**Table 1**) using the 1st generation DES – LEMANS [26], SYNTAX left main [27], BOUDRIOT [28], and PRECOMBAT trails [29].

LEMANS [26] trial is the first RCT showed PCI comparable rates of death, myocardial infarction (MI), stroke and target vessel revascularization (TVR) at 1 and 5 years with CABG for LM disease. BOUDRIOT [28] study of 100 PCI patient's v/s 101 CABG patients showed PCI was inferior to CABG at one year. In PRECOMBAT [29] trial, 600 patients randomized to LMCA PCI with first-generation drug eluting stent (DES) or CABG which showed 17.5% major adverse cerebro-cardiovascular events (MACCE) in PCI group compared to 14.3% in CABG group at 5 years of follow-up, and no significant differences in the all cause death, MI and stroke with an increased target vessel revascularization in PCI group (11.4% vs. 5.5%). At 10 years, MACCE was 29.8% in the PCI group and 24.7% in the CABG group. No significant differences were found with respect to death, stroke, or MI. However, the incidence of TVR was significantly higher in the PCI group.

A subsequent study from the French Left Main Taxus (FLM Taxus) and the Left Main with Xience (LEMAX) registries [30], comparing 2-year outcomes using either everolimus eluting stent (EES) or paclitaxel eluting stent (PES), demonstrated a reduction in target lesion failure (TLF) – a composite of cardiac death, target vessel MI, and clinically driven TLR – with PES, by 53% at 2 years (EES: 7.6% vs. PES: 16.3%,). Significant differences in target vessel MI (PES: 9.9% vs. EES: 4.1%,) and target vessel failure (PES: 16.3% vs. EES: 7.6%) were associated with EES at 2 years. Furthermore higher SYNTAX Score groups (intermediate-high) demonstrated a trend towards improved clinical benefit in patients treated with EES compared to PES.

The SYNTAX trial [27] was initially published in 2009, and it remains the landmark study for decision-making and risk stratification of complex coronary artery disease (CAD), compared TAXUS (paclitaxel coated stent) v/s CABG consisting of 1800 patients randomized to PCI with TAXUS v/s CABG in Triple Vessel Disease and LM Disease (705 patients) involving 62 EU sites and 23 US sites.

Results were analyzed according to different sub groups based on SYNTAX score (**Figure 3**) - Low SYNTAX score < 22, intermediate score > 22 - <32, and high syntax score > 32. Study showed PCI was inferior to CABG for the composite primary end points of death, MI, stroke and unplanned revascularization [31]. SYNTAX study follow up results of 1 year and 5 years showed that CABG is associated with fewer major adverse cardiac and cerebrovascular events compared with PCI. The SYNTAX

Trail	Recruitment period	N (PCI / CABG)	Longest follow-up, Y	Primary end point	Key findings	Strength	Weakness
LEMANS [26]	2001–2004	52/53	10	Change in left ventricular ejection fraction (LVEF)	Improvement in LVEF only with PCI, comparable rates of death, MI, stroke or TVR at 1 & 5 years	1st RCT comparing PCI & CABG for LM disease	Very small number of pts., surrogate primary end point, DES used only in 35%
SYNTAX-LM [27]	2005–2007	357/348	5	Death, MI, stroke or RR	PCI was non-inferior to CABG at 1 & 5 years	1st moderate sized RCT, mainly used for the current guideline recommendation	Sub-group analysis, only hypothesis generating
BOUDRIOT [28]	2003–2009	100/101	1	Cardiac death, MI or TVR	PCI was inferior to CABG at 1 year	1st RCT comparing sirolimus-eluting stents and CABG for LM disease	Limited sample size Lack of long-term follow-up, Stroke was not included in end pint
PRECOMBAT [29]	2004–2009	300/300	5	Death, MI, stroke or RR	PCI was non-inferior to CABG at 1 & 5 years	1st LM specific moderate sized RCT comparing DES & CABG for disease	Non-inferiority margin was wide, Routine angiographic follow-up in the PCI group

Table 1.
Prior trials of PCI vs CABG for LMCA in the era of the 1st generation DES.

Right dominance

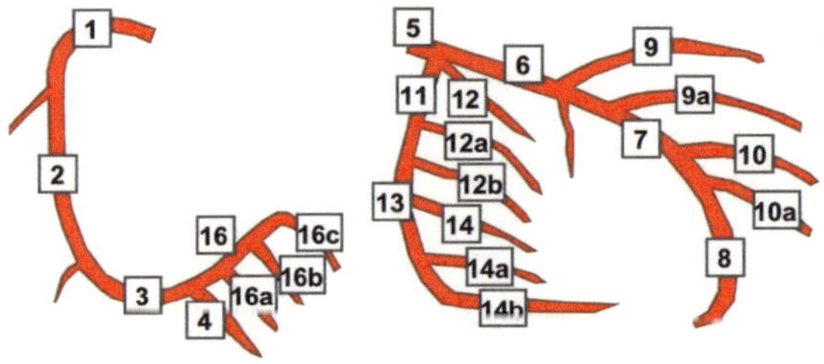

	Segment	Weighting
RCA	1, 2, 3, 4	1
	16, 16a, 16b, 16c	0.5
LMCA	5	5
LAD	6	3.5
	7	2.5
	8, 9a, 9b	1
	10, 10a	0.5
LCX	11	1.5
	12, 12a, 12b	1
	13, 14, 14a, 14b	0.5

Left dominance

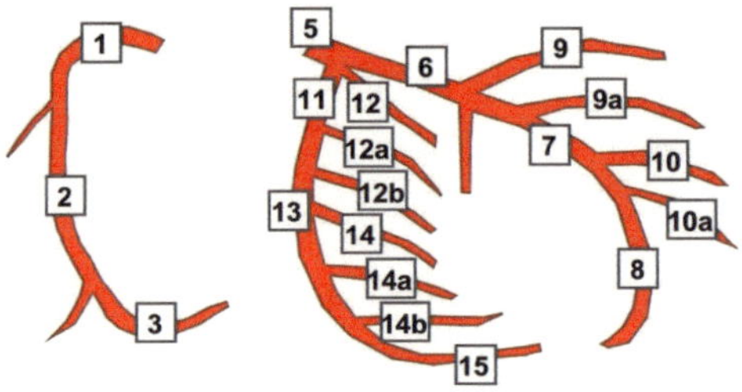

	Segment	Weighting
RCA	1, 2, 3	0
LMCA	5	6
LAD	6	3.5
	7	2.5
	8, 9a, 9b	1
	10, 10a	0.5
LCX	11	2.5
	12, 12a, 12b	1
	13	1.5
	14, 14a, 14b, 15	1

Figure 3.
Coronary segment weighting derived from Leamon score.

study emphasized the heart team concept and the SYNTAX score to assess the risk status by grading of the patients' coronary disease burden. SYNTAX LM subset consisting of low and intermediate score 0–32 showed similar cumulative event rate 32.1% and 31.3% in CABG group v/s TAXUS group at 5 years follow-up and higher cumulative event rate at 5 years follow up in CABG compared to PCI 46.5% v/s 29.7% in LM subset with high SYNTAX SCORE > 33, and results demonstrated that surgery remains the gold standard for patients with complex multi vessel disease. 2009 American college of cardiology (ACC)/American heart association (AHA) guidelines recommended PCI of LMCA class II–b for noncomplex LMCA disease based on meta-analysis of multiple trails among patients with 1st generation DES showed that death, MI and stroke (major adverse cardiac events - MACE) were starting to show similarity in PCI and CABG patients at 1 year.

SYNTAX score guides in assessing severity and extent of CAD and provides information to take proper decision in planning appropriate revascularization strategy. The clinical SYNTAX score is a combination of age, creatinine and ejection fraction (ACEF) model and SYNTAX scores, and subsequent development of a logistic model has provided better risk assessment [31]. The SYNTAX II score is useful to predicts long-term mortality in patients with severe triple-vessel or LMCA disease, and it is assessed by considering anatomical and clinical factors (age, creatinine clearance, LV function, gender, chronic obstructive pulmonary disease, and peripheral vascular disease) along with SYNTAX score. It was found to be superior to the conventional SYNTAX score in guiding decision-making between CABG and PCI in the risk assessment. The STS (The Society of Thoracic Surgeons) score is a risk-prediction model, validated in patients undergoing cardiac surgery, with a specific model for CABG and combined CABG and valve surgery. It can be used to predict in-hospital or 30-day mortality and in-hospital morbidity [32]. ACCF/AHA guideline suggests that calculation of the SYNTAX and STS scores is reasonable in patients with unprotected LM and complex CAD (Class IIa recommendation, level of evidence; B).

The DELTA registry (n = 2,775), [33] a multi-center, multinational registry of LM PCI with first generation DES (n = 1,874, PES or SES) against CABG (n = 901) for ULMCA disease, no differences in the primary composite endpoint of all-cause death, CVA and MI were seen (HR 1.11; 95% CI 0.85–1.42; p = 0.47).

2.7 Experience of PCI of LMCA with 2nd generation DES

EXCEL [34] and NOBLE [35] are the two major trials to see efficacy of 2nd generation DES v/s CABG based on the evidence of superior results of 2nd Generation Everolimus drug eluting (XIENCE) in reducing MACE rate against TAXUS in SPRIT III and CIPHER in ISAR-test 4 trail with a lower mortality rate (22%) at 10 years. Unfavorable results reported in some trails of PCI of LMCA lesions may be due to use of earlier generation stents and to various technical issues such as catheter induced dissections, under expansion, uncovered diseased segments, multiple mal apposed stent layers, jailing of Ostium multiple struts, longitudinal compression of struts and accidentally crushed stent which will contribute to worse out comes .Similarly, many advances took place in the field of CABG by total arterial revascularization using left internal mammary artery (LIMA), right internal mammary artery (RIMA), and bilateral internal mammary artery (BIMA), on pump v/s off pump Bypass surgery, minimally invasive techniques, sternal sparing, endovascular harvesting, and hybrid philosophy.

The EXCEL trial [34] was a prospective randomized open-label, non-inferiority trial undertaken at 126 centers in 17 countries around the world. Study included 948 patients XIENCE group v/s CABG 957 patients with unprotected LMCA with >70% DS, or > 50–70% with either 1) Non-invasive evidence of LM ischemia, 2) IVUS MLA < 6.0 mm^2, or 3) FFR: <0.80 with SYNTAX SCORE < 32. SYNTAX score was ≤22 in 60.5%, >23 – <32 in 39.5%, and distal LMCA was present in 80.5% of the patients. IVUS guidance was used in nearly 80% of the patients in the PCI group. It included both stable and unstable angina but excluded patients of ST elevation myocardial infarction (STEMI). Distal bifurcating lesions were treated with a two-stent strategy using various techniques. CABG was performed both on- and off-pump, with the aim of complete revascularization for vessels with 50% stenosis. There was no difference between the two groups in respect to the primary composite end-point event of death, stroke, or myocardial infarction at 3 years (15.4% of the patients in the PCI group and in 14.7% of the patients in the CABG group), ischemia-driven revascularization was more frequent after PCI compared to CABG (in 12.6% vs. 7.5% of the patients, p < 0.001), and Stent thrombosis occurred in only 0.7% of patients within 3 years which was less common than symptomatic graft occlusion. EXCEL 5 years follow-up data showed primary end point - All cause death, stroke or MI 22.9% in PCI group v/s 19.2% in CABG group. In EXCEL study [34] IVUS use was not mandatory which was used in only 77% of patients, and no specific bifurcation technique was followed which was left to the operator discretion, and the use of proximal optimization technique (POT) and final kissing balloon (FKB) were also not specified (**Table 2**), these would have influenced study outcomes.

The Nordic-Baltic-British Left Main Revascularization Study [35] is a prospective, randomized, open-label, non-inferiority trial done at 36 centers in Europe. Patients with

Recommendations according to extent of CAD	CABG		PCI	
	Class	Level	Class	Level
Left main CAD				
Left main disease with low SYNTAX score (0–22)	I	A	I	A
Left main disease with intermediate SYNTAX score (23–32)	I	A	IIa	A
Left main disease with high SYNTAX score (≥ 33)	I	A	III	B

Table 2.
Recommendations for the type of revascularization with left main disease.

LMCA visually assessed with diameter ≥ 50% or fractional flow reserve ≤0.80 in different segments of the left main coronary artery were randomized to CABG or PCI with Biolimus eluting stent. SYNTAX score was calculated and all patients with low, medium, and high score were included. Patients were treated with the intention of achieving complete revascularization (CR). Distal LM bifurcation was treated with "Culotte" technique in majority of patients, enrolled 592 patients in each group, on-pump CABG was performed in 84% of patients, and LIMA graft was used in 96% of patients. Results showed higher MACCE rate in PCI group (28%) compared to CABG (18%) group due to higher MI and repeat revascularization in PCI group, but without significant difference in overall mortality and stroke rate. PCI group experienced lower stroke rate at 30 days of follow up compared to CABG group, but this difference was not seen at 1- and 5-year follow-up. In NOBLE study, only 75% underwent IVUS, FKB was performed in 55% of patients, 8% were implanted with first generation DES, and these factors might have influenced study outcomes to some extent.

2.8 Meta-analysis of PCI vs CABG

Individual patient data analysis from 11 PCI v/s CABG trails consisting of 11,518 randomized patients out of which, 4,394 (38.9%) (**Figure 4**) patients with LM disease showed all-cause mortality of 10.7% in CABG patient v/s 10.7% in PCI patients at follow-up of 5 years' period which also showed mortality after LM DES v/s CABG 12.8 v/s 14.6% in SYNTAX, 5.7% v/s 7.9% in PRECOMBAT, 13.0% v/s 9.9% in EXCEL and 9.4% vs. 8.7% in NOBLE studies. Higher all-cause mortality was observed in PCI group v/s CABG in LM subset patients with diabetes 16.5% v/s 13.5% and patients with syntax score > 32–15% v/s 12.4% [35].

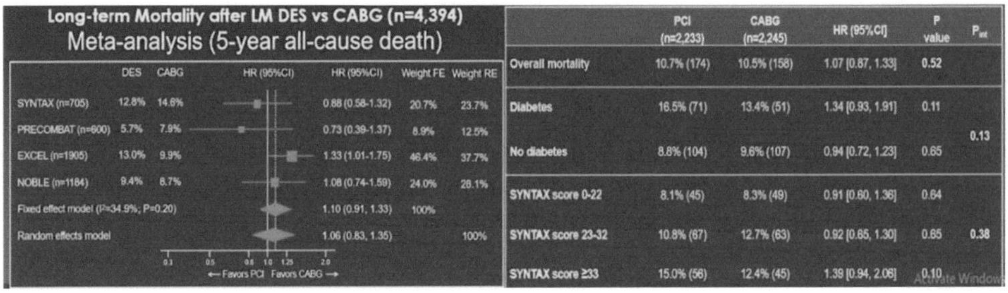

Figure 4.
Meta-analysis of PCI vs CABG.

2.9 Long term evidence of PCI of LMCA with DES

LM registry analysis of a total of 913 patients who underwent LM PCI at FU- WAI hospital between 2004 to 2008 revealed ten year outcomes of unprotected LM PCI in selected patients had acceptable results, though majority were implanted with 1st generation DES, and reduced 10 years mortality of PCI of LM was observed in lower risk patients stratified by SYNTAX Score and SYNTAX II, IVUS guidance, and usage of DES can significantly reduce 10 years mortality, stroke, and MI. Study suggested Age, LV EF, and incomplete revascularization are independent predictors of 10 years death or MI [36].

MAIN COMPARE Study of LMCA stenting v/s CABG showed The rate of target vessel failure (TVF), risk of death, and serious composite outcomes higher in PCI compared to CABG after 5 years [37] & 10 years [38] follow up results showed no significant difference in the rates of death and composite end points of death, Q wave MI and stroke between PCI and CABG groups.

The **SYNTAXES** study (Synergy Between Percutaneous Coronary Intervention with TAXUS and Cardiac Surgery Extended Survival) is the 10-year follow-up of the original SYNTAX trial [39], comprising 72% of the syntax 10 years' data (No: 1301), showed a comparable survival rate between CABG group 26.7% and PCI group 26.1% at 10 years (**Figure** 5).

2.10 Evidence of PCI vs CABG for ostial and shaft LMCA

Meta-analysis of studies comparing the clinical outcome (MACE) in 3291 patients receiving PCI with DES stenting of Ostial & Mid shaft showed favorable outcome compared with distal LM lesions. Excel study also revealed better 3 years' outcome (Death, MI or Stroke) after Ostial and shaft lesions of LM (CABG 13.5% v/s PCI 12.4%) compared with LM bifurcation v/s CABG (CABG 14.9% v/s 15.6% PCI) [34].

2.11 General principles of PCI of LMCA

PCI of LM is a high risk interventional procedure requires meticulous planning, adequate skills and experience to produce best possible results. PCI of ostium and

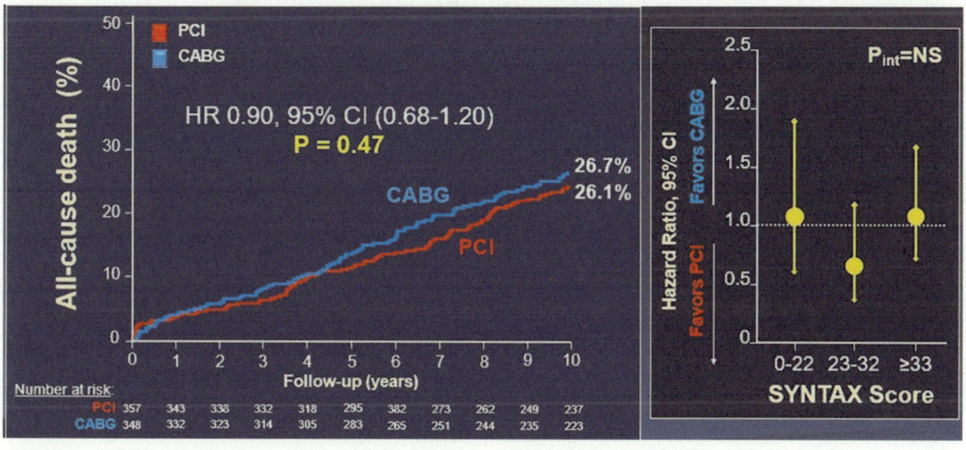

Figure 5.
SYNTAX left Main at 10 years: Mortality.

shaft carries better results compared to LM bifurcation. PCI of distal LM associated with more risk and increased MACE due to requirement of more number of stents in complex lesions, and tendency for increased restenosis at ostium of LCX.

High risk may be due to associated co-morbidities, complex coronary anatomy and hemodynamic compromise status. Most of the patients undergoing LM PCI do not require hemodynamic support, but the operator should consider it if he anticipates or encounters any hemodynamic compromise, slow or no reflow or other procedural complications (**Figure 6**). During pre-procedure evaluation of LMCA revascularization screen for its association with carotid artery disease, cerebrovascular disease and peripheral artery disease, aortic aneurysm, and porcelain aorta which make the surgical procedure more challenging. Compared to unprotected lesions, complications of PCI (abrupt closure and restenosis) of protected LMCA lesions are more often well tolerated because of continued flow to the protected territory [40]. Significant LMCA disease more often associated with Carotid artery disease which is seen in nearly 40% of patients undergoing angiography for angina. The AHA guidelines recommend screening of all patients undergoing bypass surgery for left main stem disease to identify carotid artery disease [41].

Take precautions to reduce contrast volume to avoid contrast induced nephropathy (CIN) and exposure to radiation while performing high-risk, complex LM PCI. Use appropriate devices to expedite the procedure by using guide extension catheters, adequate guide catheter backs up for good support, micro catheters, guide wires, balloons to avoid complications related to procedure delay, and use standard current generation DES for best possible results. It would be preferable to keep thin profile balloons to cross critical lesions, high pressure balloons, and scoring balloons to tackle tough un-dilatable lesions which are difficult to dilate with regular NC balloons to improve procedural success and long term outcomes.

2.12 Advantages of PCI over CABG

PCI is less invasive with fewer peri -procedural complications, fewer 30 day MACE, early rapid recovery with better quality of life (QOL) and earlier angina relief. It is preferable in patients who require urgent revascularizations mainly in ACS setting, coexisting serious co-morbidities and comes under high surgical risk (ie., chronic lung disease, advanced age, history of previous stroke, and prior Bypass surgery).

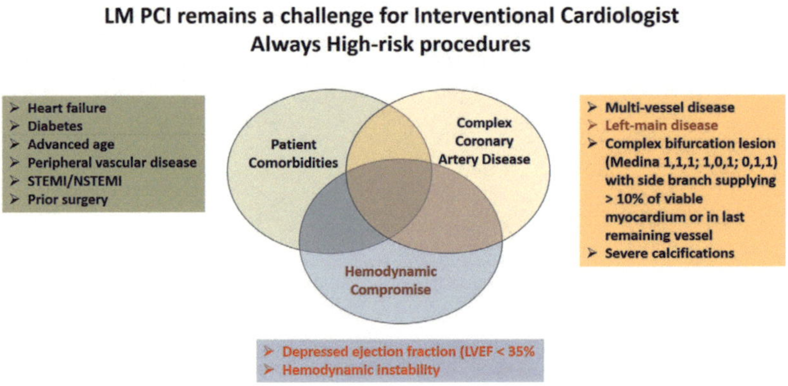

Figure 6.
Challenges for LM PCI for interventional cardiologists in high-risk procedures.

2.13 Revascularization strategy of angiographically significant LMCA disease during Acute STEMI-PCI vs CABG

Revascularization of Acute STEMI patients with significant LM lesions depends upon the culprit vessel, type of MI, dominant vessel, complexity of coronary disease and anatomy, and hemodynamic status. In patients with Acute Inferior STEMI with significant LM (non-culprit) with multi vessel disease, and culprit vessel is right coronary artery (RCA), recommended to perform primary PCI of culprit vessel only with optimal medical therapy for bystander lesions and PCI/CABG of the non-culprit arteries only for spontaneous angina or myocardial ischaemia on stress testing or LM with multi-vessel (MV) PCI guided by angiography or FFR after finishing culprit PCI during same sitting. Primary PCI of Culprit vessel only, followed by angiography or FFR-driven staged PCI of non-culprit arteries during the index hospitalization or after hospital discharge.

Acute STEMI with cardiogenic shock – Recommended to perform culprit vessel PCI initially, then PCI of LM and other vessels is reasonable option if no improvement in hemodynamic status but should be differed if hemodynamic status improves after culprit PCI (**Figure** 7). If culprit vessel is LAD or LCX in STEMI patients with significant LM disease, consider PCI of LM along with PCI of LAD or LCX. If the patient is having STEMI with LM and multi-vessel disease (MVD), perform Primary PCI of culprit vessel, and if the non-culprit vessel or vessels are having significant disease (>70% stenosis), complete the revascularization of all diseased vessels during original hospital stay. If the non-culprit lesion has intermediate lesion (40–70% stenosis), perform PCI of non-culprit lesions under FFR/ iFR guidance or 5–7 days after massive MI.

2.14 Early vs Delayed CABG in Acute STEMI

Early CABG is associated with mortality rate (MR) in acute MI, preferable to postpone surgery for 3 to 5 days in the absence of absolute indications for CABG due to high mortality rate with very early surgery. Multicenter study of 32,099 cases

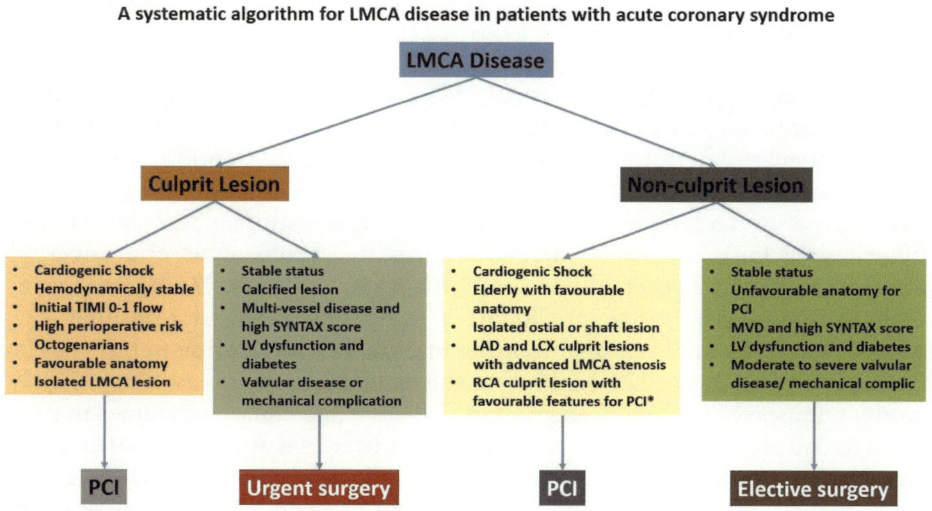

Figure 7.
A systemic algorithm for LMCA disease in patients with ACS.

reported by Lee and colleagues, showed mortality rate of 14.2% if operated within 6 hours, vs. 2.7% if operated beyond 15 days [42]. Thielmann et.al reported mortality rate of 23.8% if operated between 7 and 24 hours, and 2.4% if operated between 8 to 14 days period [43]. Early CABG in STEMI is associated with reduction in the size of infarct, and reduces the potential for mechanical complications whereas late CABG associated with reperfusion injury and increased systemic inflammatory response syndrome (SIRS).

In STEMI and multi vessel disease associated with cardiogenic shock short-term mechanical support device (e.g., percutaneous cardiopulmonary support, extra corporeal membrane oxygenation (ECMO), or ventricular assist device) with / without intra-aortic balloon pump (IABP) may be considered as a rescue therapy in patients with refractory circulatory support.

2.15 Hemodynamic support during LM PCI

Mechanical circulatory support devices should be considered while performing high risk LM interventions particularly in the presence of severe LV dysfunction, unstable status hemodynamic status reflected by left ventricular end diastolic pressure (LVEDP) >20 mm Hg, systolic BP <100 mm Hg, or mixed venous oxygen saturation < 55%, and complex procedures requiring longer time specially while handling diffusely calcified multi vessel disease, or single surviving vessel to avoid sudden hemodynamic collapse which might result in stoppage of procedure in midway, or might not get enough time to carry effective cardiopulmonary resuscitation (CPR) to revive the patient.

2.16 Influence of stenting technique and optimization on LM PCI outcomes

Provisional stenting is the technique of choice in bifurcation lesions, as it is technically simpler with improved clinical outcomes to a systematic 2-stent strategy. Many Bifurcation trials like NORDIC [44], BBC ONE [45], BBK [46], CACTUS [47] have not shown any benefit associated with systematic two-stent strategies, and EBC TWO study [48] also showed worse outcomes with systematic dual stenting even in patients with larger, true bifurcations. Ample evidence from non-randomized trials showing worse outcomes for two-stent techniques. However, randomized data from Dr. Shao-Liang Chen et al. support Double Kissing (DK)-crush in left main bifurcations Patients with true bifurcation should be treated with two stents preferably with DKC, because of recent evidence of better results, compared to provisional stenting, and other two stent techniques [49]. DKCRUSH II showed that a 2-stent strategy using the double kissing (DK) crush technique is superior to provisional stenting particularly in more complex lesions [50]. DKCRUSH-III, showed superior results of DK crush over Coulotte technique at 3 years with lower MACCE rate (8.2% vs. 23.7%) and stent thrombosis (0% vs. 3.7%) [51]. DKCRUSH-V study showed superior results DK crush technique compared to provisional stenting in distal LM bifurcation in terms of lower TLF at 1 year (5% versus 10.7%) and stent thrombosis (0.4% versus 3.3%) [52]. Recently, published EBC MAIN was designed to examine clinical outcomes in patients are treated equally well with a stepwise layered provisional approach, starting with a single stent, as with a more complex dual stent implant, and Only one-fifth of patients in provisional group required second stent showed Procedure time, X-ray dose and consumables were less, fewer adverse events systematic provisional (n-230) vs. systematic dual approach (n – 237) with a MACE rate of 14.7% vs. 17.7%,

Death 3%vs. 4.2%, MI 10% vs10.1%, TLR 6.1% vs. 9.3%, and stent thrombosis (ST) 1.7% vs. 1.3%, they concluded that The stepwise provisional strategy should remain the approach of choice for the majority of left main bifurcation interventions [53]. Angio graphic ISR more frequent in lesions with under-expansion than without (24.1% Vs 5.4%), and proper use of kissing balloon and POT is essential to get the good expansion and proper opposition of stent struts. In the 2 stent group, the lesions with complete expansion of all sites showed a restenosis of only 6%, similar to that in the single stent group (6.3%). It would be preferable to achieve post bifurcation PCI MSA of LM > 8 mm^2, LM confluence >7mm^2, LAD ostium >6mm^2 and LCX ostium >5mm^2 or aim to achieve mean reference diameter of stented area at least >80% compared to proximal and distal reference areas. Post-stenting under-expansion was an independent predictor of 2-year MACE, especially repeat revascularization (**Figure 8**).

Intravascular imaging and FFR should be used to optimize DES results, to stent only physiologically significant lesions, to avoid unnecessary stenting thereby reduces number of stents. Kang et al. evaluated IVUS predictors of ISR after LM bifurcation stenting, and post-stenting IVUS mean stent area (MSA) cut-offs that best predicted ISR on a segmental basis were 5.0 mm^2 (ostial LCX), 6.3 mm^2 (ostial LAD), 7.2 mm^2 (POC, confluence zone of LAD and LCX), and 8.2 mm^2 (LM above the POC). A smaller IVUS-MSA within any one of these segments was responsible for a higher rate of angiographic ISR and clinical major adverse cardiovascular events (MACE) [54].

IVUS guided PCI of LM stenting associated with trend towards decreased mortality that is 13.6% v/s 6.0%. ADAPT – DES [55] study and ULTIMATE study [56], and recent IVUS meta-analysis also highlighted the same, implement the optimal stenting techniques and optimize DES implantation with IVI to provide best acute and long term results.

2.17 CABG vs PCI of LMCA in diabetics

CABG is the standard revascularization strategy in patients with diabetes mellitus (DM) and multi-vessel or complex CAD with long term favorable outcomes. Recent evidence suggests that PCI is a safe and effective modality for patients with LMCA

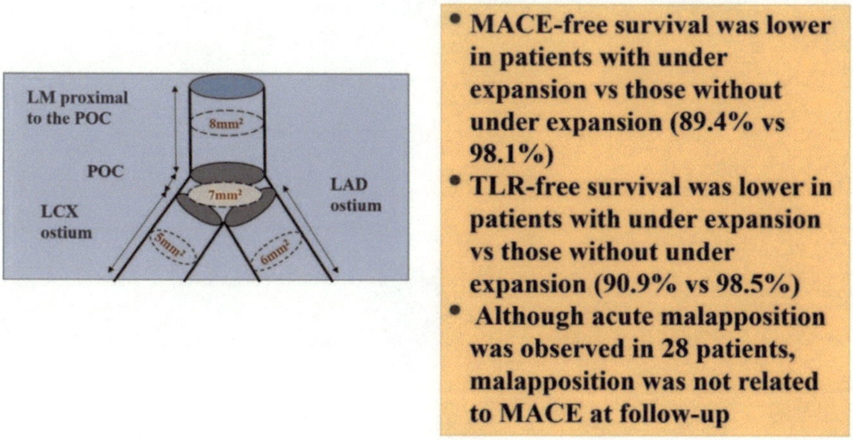

Figure 8.
Criteria for stent under-expansion at the distal LMCA bifurcation.

disease with <22 and > 22 to <32 syntax score as compared with CABG, no significant difference in the 10-year risks of mortality and serious composite outcome after PCI or CABG in patients both with and without DM, but the risk of TVR was consistently higher after PCI. In a recent pooled analysis of individual patient data, the presence of DM was reported to have a significant interaction effect for 5-year mortality favoring CABG over PCI in patients with multi-vessel CAD, but not in those with LMCA disease. These findings also confirmed the impact of DM with respect to the primary composite end point and mortality in the subgroup analysis of the EXCEL trial with low to intermediate SYNTAX scores.

The FREEDOM trial 8 years' follow-up data showed that CABG leads to lower all-cause mortality than PCI in patients with DM with multi vessel disease [57]. The benefit of CABG in patients with DM might be attributed to complete revascularization in more diffuse and complex multi vessel CAD. By contrast, moving on to the DES era, DM did not appear to modify the treatment effects of PCI and CABG for LMCA disease.

2.18 Influence of Hospital and operator volume on LM PCI outcomes

Hospital and operator volume also impacts the outcomes of LMCA PCI, and results are better in a center with a high volume and operated by high volume operator (**Figure 9**), all cause death (0.5% v/s 2.1%) and cardiac death (0.5 v/s 2.1%). Study revealed that results are better with the operators who were performing at least 15 PCI of LMCA per year in 3 consecutive years [58].

2.19 Heart team approach – Risk assessment of CABG vs PCI

LM PCI out comes can be improved with the proper selection of patients after assessing risk v/s benefit by involving Heart team with adequate counseling and education about decease nature and various modes of treatment options. All patients with LM disease should be assessed with SYNTAX, Functional SYNTAX, SYNTAX II, EURO & STS scores (**Table 3**) to assess risk and mortality rate and to decide plan of treatment

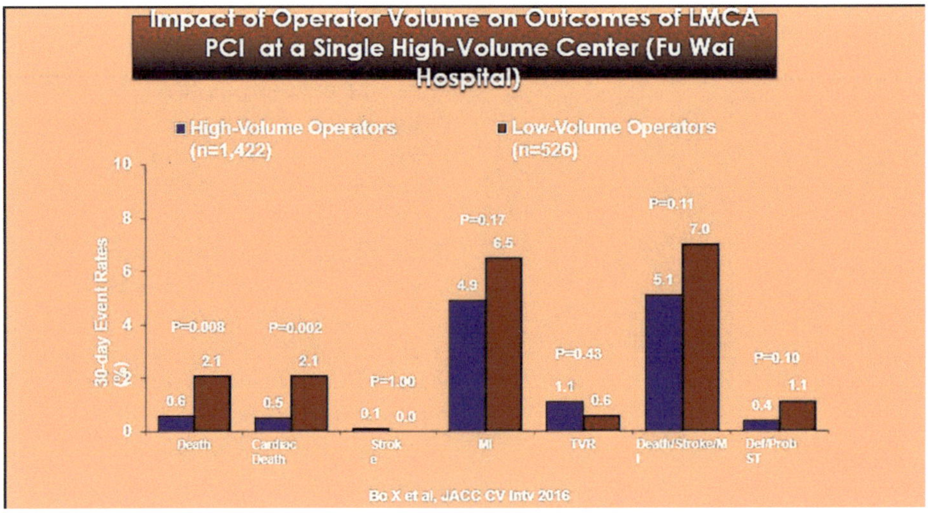

Figure 9.
Impact of operator volume on outcomes of LMCA PCI.

Recommendations:	**Class**	**Level**
Assessment of surgical risk		
It is recommended that the STS score is calculated to assess in-hospital or 30 day mortality, and in-hospital mortality after CABG	I	B
Calculation of the EuroSCORE II score may be considered to assess in-hospital mortality after CABG	IIb	B
Assessment of CAD complexity		
In patients with LM or multi-vessel disease, it is recommended that the SYNTAX score is calculated to assess the anatomical complexity of CAD and the long-term risk of mortality and morbidity after PCI	I	B
When considering the decision between CABG and PCI, completeness of revascularization should be prioritized	IIa	B
PCI should be considered, if the Heart Team is concerned about the surgical risk or if the patient refuses CABG after adequate counseling by the Heart Team.		

Table 3.
Criteria for the choice between PCI and CABG.

involving Heart team. The most widely used surgical risk score is the Society of Thoracic Surgeons score. It classifies operative risk based on predicted risk of mortality into low (<4%), intermediate (4% to <8%), high (8% to <12%), or extreme (≥12%). The newly incorporated "Functional SYNTAX score" (Functional SXscore) essentially incorporates FFR measurements into the SYNTAX Score calculation, and was recently shown potentially to improve the stratification of low and high risk patients, when compared to the conventional visual-based angiographic approach [59]. The heart team should assess risks and benefits of surgery in the high- and extreme-risk population, and careful evaluation of clinical history, physical examination for co-morbidities with necessary investigations to plan for appropriate revascularization strategies after proper and repeated counseling of the patient and his or her relatives. Special attention should be focused on frailty, cognitive status, acute and long term results, importance of life style modification including stopping of smoking and long term usage and adherence of drug therapy to control risk factors and to prevent recurrence of angina and MI from progression of atheroma in grafts and native vessels.

Currently, in the US guidelines (**Table 2**), PCI has a class IIa recommendation ("is reasonable") in select patients with isolated LM stenosis involving the ostium or shaft and without coexisting multi vessel disease and the risk of surgical bypass is increased. PCI has a class IIb recommendation ("may be reasonable") in patients with LM stenosis involving the distal bifurcation or with less complex coexisting multi vessel disease as defined by a low or intermediate SYNTAX score (≤33) and who have an elevated surgical risk. The current US guidelines recommend against PCI in patients who are good candidates for surgical bypass with coexisting complex multi vessel disease as defined by highest tertile of the SYNTAX score (≥33). Hybrid bypass is another revascularization approach m that combines coronary bypass using a minimally invasive direct coronary artery bypass approach of grafting the LIMA to LAD artery and PCI to the remaining vessels in an attempt to achieve the most desired aspects of each revascularization strategy. Always aim for complete revascularization because major adverse cardiovascular events including mortality are higher in patients with incomplete revascularization than those with complete revascularization regardless of the revascularization strategy.

2.20 Who should be treated with CABG?

CABG has more durable long term outcome with fewer adverse events beyond 30 days particularly MI due to protection against future events, improved long term relief of angina and repeat revascularization procedures particularly in more complex anatomies more often due to complete revascularization. It is preferred in patients with poor LV function, long standing DM, concomitant cardiac surgery, high bleeding risk patients who are unable to comply with dual anti-platelet therapy (DAPT). CABG scores over PCI in patients with LM with addition Triple Vessel Disease, unsuitable for PCI due to complex anatomy, severely calcified and tortuous of coronaries, chronic total occlusion (CTO), Multiple diffuse long segment lesions, and complex ISR lesions. Patients with critical LMCA disease with severe symptoms or with life-threatening ventricular arrhythmias, which is believed to be ischemic in origin should be subjected for early surgery because of increased incidence of sudden death. CABG surgery associated with in hospital mortality rate of 1%, and < 3% perioperative MI in low-risk patients Surgery associated with increased incidence of Peri -operative MI, bleeding and transfusions, arrhythmias, renal failure, increased incidence of sternal dehiscence, and Repeat revascularization. Predictors of increased mortality after CABG are emergency procedure, extreme age, past history of cardiac surgery, female gender, LV dysfunction, severity of LM stenosis, and number of vessels with significant stenosis.

2.21 On pump vs off pump CABG

CABG with on-pump surgery considered as a preferred and standard revascularization procedure for 80% of CAD patients after seeing successful results of series of surgical cases following first CABG in the late 1960s. On-pump surgery has problems related to manipulation of the ascending aorta leading cerebrovascular accidents particularly in patients with aotic-atheroma and porcelain aorta, myo-necrosis due to aortic occlusion, cognitive dysfunction, renal failure, and systemic inflammatory response syndrome. Whereas, off-pump surgical technique overcomes these limitations, and is more often associated with hemodynamic instability, mainly in patients with recent MI, LV dysfunction, dilated ventricles, and while grafting the branches of the LCx in patients with significant mitral insufficiency, and less complete revascularization. Compared to traditional on-pump CABG with LIMA to LAD, irrespective of SVG or arterial grafts to other vessels neither off-pump CABG nor the use of bilateral internal mammary arteries has been shown to improve CABG outcomes in RCTs.

2.22 Influence of arterial vs venous grafts on long term outcomes of CABG

Advantages of CABG over PCI - PCI treats an isolated lesion in the proximal vessel, complexity of the lesion affects clinical outcome, CABG by passes the proximal 2/3 of the vessel, where current lesions and future threatening lesions can occur. This advantage will persist, even if stent restenosis is zero. The LIMA is the ideal graft of choice to bypass the LAD artery (Class I recommendation for ACCF/AHA guideline for CABG surgery) due to graft patency of LIMA is >90% after 10 years. LIMA is resistant to atherosclerosis, and release prostacyclin and nitric oxide contributing to vasodilation, inhibition of platelet function, and improved survival rate which is independent of the patient's sex, age, extent of CAD, and LV systolic function. LIMA to LAD graft decreases the occurrence of late MI, reoperation, recurrence of angina, and repeated hospitalizations. Radial artery graft patency results are better when it is grafted to Lcx with >70% narrowing and worst when it is used to graft the RCA with a stenosis of only moderate severity. Patency of Radial artery grafts better when used for >90% lesions, and choose the radial artery of non-dominant upper-limb, and radial artery with a > 2 mm diameter after testing modified Allen test for ulnar dominance. Combination of LIMA, RIMA, radial artery, and or gastroepiploic artery may be used for full arterial revascularization processes. Reversed saphenous vein grafts are also routinely used in combination with LIMA, RIMA, and other arterial grafts in patients undergoing CABG surgery depending upon suitability of grafts. Saphenous vein grafts (SVG) have a track record of poor long-term patency with a closure rate of about 10–25% during 1st year post CABG period, an additional closure rate of 1–2% each year during the 1–5 years of post-surgery, and 4–5% occlude each year between 6 and 10 years postoperatively, with an overall 10 years' patency of SVGs is about 50–60%. Major determinants of graft selection are age, severity of narrowing of the vessel and hemodynamic status of the patient. LIMA-LAD graft should be offered to all patients with LMCA disease undergoing CABG either with on-pump or off-pump with aim of total revascularization.

2.23 Post CABG progression of atherosclerosis

Post CABG patients develops progression of atherosclerosis in native vessels which was accelerated by vein grafts and observed in over 50% of the native vessels, 35% of native coronary arteries bypassed with a venous grafts progressed to total occlusion in 35% of SVG compared to 8% of LIMA. Vein graft failure associated with increased death, MI and revascularization.

2.24 Adjunctive Therapy and supportive measures for LM disease

All patients with LMCA with or without revascularization should be emphasized about the need to continue adequate guideline directed therapies such as DAPT, anti-Hypertensive (calcium channel blockers (CCB), angiotensin converting enzyme inhibitors (ACEI), angiotensin receptor blockers (ARB), and beta blockers (BB)), anti-Diabetic drugs (SGL2 inhibitors, and Metformin), high dose statin therapy, and drugs for LV Dysfunction (ARNIs, SGL2 inhibitors, aldosterone antagonists, and beta blockers) to provide better long term results of revascularization. Patients with poly vascular disease should be recommended with Rivaroxaban 2.5 mg bid, and aspirin 100 mg, diabetics with renal dysfunction and heart failure should be supplemented with SGL2 inhibitors to reduce repeat hospitalizations, and MACE rates. During follow up all patients should be monitored for any recurrence of symptoms which requires appropriate evaluation with necessary investigations and adequate control of risk factors and life style modification.

3. Conclusion

Angiographic assessment of borderline LM lesions (30–70%) is inaccurate with significant inter-observer variability.1 Intravascular imaging is helpful in assessing severity and to decide revascularization strategies particularly in patients with angiography showing lesions of uncertain severity, and recent evidence is in more favor of image guided PCI over angio guided PCI with improved clinical outcomes.

Acknowledgements

The author would like to thank Mr. Manikandhar Pendyala and Mr. Chandrashekar Challa for their assistance in the manuscript preparation.

Author details

Sridhar Kasturi
Department and Senior Interventional Cardiologist, Sunshine Hospitals, Secunderabad, Telangana, India

*Address all correspondence to: sridharkasturi@yahoo.com

References

[1] Villa AD, Sammut E, Nair A, Rajani R, Bonamini R, Chiribiri A. Coronary artery anomalies overview: The normal and the abnormal. World Journal of Radiology. 2016;**8**(6):537

[2] Park SJ, Park DW. Percutaneous coronary intervention with stent implantation versus coronary artery bypass surgery for treatment of left main coronary artery disease: Is it time to change guidelines? Circulation: Cardiovascular Interventions. 2009;**2**(1):59-68

[3] Stary HC, Chandler AB, Dinsmore RE, Fuster V, Glagov S, Insull W Jr, et al. A definition of advanced types of atherosclerotic lesions and a histological classification of atherosclerosis: A report from the Committee on Vascular Lesions of the Council on Arteriosclerosis. American Heart Association. Circulation. 1995; **92**(5):1355-1374

[4] Gould KL, Kirkeeide RL, Buchi M. Coronary flow reserve as a physiologic measure of stenosis severity. Journal of the American College of Cardiology. 1990;**15**(2):459-474

[5] Sanchis-Gomar F, Perez-Quilis C, Leischik R, Lucia A. Epidemiology of coronary heart disease and acute coronary syndrome. Annals of Translational Medicine. 2016;**4**(13):1-12

[6] Oviedo C, Maehara A, Mintz GS, Araki H, Choi SY, Tsujita K, et al. Intravascular ultrasound classification of plaque distribution in left main coronary artery bifurcations: Where is the plaque really located? Circulation: Cardiovascular Interventions. 2010;**3**(2):105

[7] Fathala A. Myocardial perfusion scintigraphy: Techniques, interpretation, indications and reporting. Annals of Saudi medicine. 2011;**31**(6):625-634

[8] Chen ML, Mo YH, Wang YC, Lo HS, Wang PC, Chao IM, et al. 64-slice CT angiography for the detection of functionally significant coronary stenoses: Comparison with stress myocardial perfusion imaging. The British Journal of Radiology. 2012; **85**(1012):368-376

[9] Koo BK, Erglis A, Doh JH, Daniels DV, Jegere S, Kim HS, et al. Diagnosis of ischemia-causing coronary stenoses by noninvasive fractional flow reserve computed from coronary computed tomographic angiograms: Results from the prospective multicenter DISCOVER-FLOW (Diagnosis of Ischemia-Causing Stenoses Obtained Via Noninvasive Fractional Flow Reserve) study. Journal of the American College of Cardiology. 2011;**58**(19):1989-1997

[10] Finet G, Huo Y, Rioufol G, Ohayon J, Guerin P, Kassab GS. Structure-function relation in the coronary artery tree: Ffluid dynamics to arterial bifurcations. EuroIntervention. 2010;**6**:419

[11] Murray CD. The physiological principle of minimum work applied to the angle of branching of arteries. The Journal of General Physiology. 1926;**9**(6):835

[12] Ramadan R, Boden WE, Kinlay S. Management of left main coronary artery disease. Journal of the American Heart Association. 2018;**7**(7):e008151

[13] Kasturi S. Current status of intra-vascular imaging during coronary interventions. World Journal of Cardiovascular Diseases. 2021;**11**(8):389-419

[14] de la Torre Hernandez JM, Hernández Hernandez F, Alfonso F,

Rumoroso JR, Lopez-Palop R, Sadaba M, et al. Prospective application of pre-defined intravascular ultrasound criteria for assessment of intermediate left main coronary artery lesions: Results from the multicenter LITRO study. Journal of the American College of Cardiology. 2011; **58**(4):351-358

[15] Park SJ, Ahn JM, Kang SJ, Yoon SH, Koo BK, Lee JY, et al. Intravascular ultrasound-derived minimal lumen area criteria for functionally significant left main coronary artery stenosis. JACC: Cardiovascular Interventions. 2014;**7**(8): 868-874

[16] Berry C, McClure JD, Oldroyd KG. Meta-analysis of death and myocardial infarction in the DEFINE-FLAIR and iFR-SWEDEHEART trials. Circulation. 2017;**136**(24):2389-2391

[17] VA Coronary Artery Bypass Surgery Cooperative Study Group. Eighteen-year follow-up in the Veterans Affairs Cooperative Study of Coronary Artery Bypass Surgery for stable angina. Circulation. 1992;**86**(1):121-130

[18] European Coronary Surgery Study Group. Prospective Randomised study of coronary artery bypass surgery in stable angina pectoris: Second Interim Report by the. The Lancet. 1980;**316**(8193):491-495

[19] Fisher LD, Judkins MP, Lesperance J, Cameron A, Swaye P, Ryan T, et al. Reproducibility of coronary arteriographic reading in the coronary artery surgery study (CASS). Catheterization and Cardiovascular Diagnosis. 1982;**8**(6):565-575

[20] Takaro T, Peduzzi P, Detre KM, Hultgren HN, Murphy ML, Van der Bel-Kahn J, et al. Survival in subgroups of patients with left main coronary artery disease. Veterans Administration Cooperative Study of Surgery for Coronary Arterial Occlusive Disease. Circulation. 1982;**66**(1):14-22

[21] O'Keefe JH Jr, Hartzler GO, Rutherford BD, McConahay DR, Johnson WL, Giorgi LV, et al. Left main coronary angioplasty: Early and late results of 127 acute and elective procedures. The American Journal of Cardiology. 1989;**64**(3):144-147

[22] Yusuf S, Zucker D, Passamani E, Peduzzi P, Takaro T, Fisher LD, et al. Effect of coronary artery bypass graft surgery on survival: Overview of 10-year results from randomised trials by the Coronary Artery Bypass Graft Surgery Trialists Collaboration. The Lancet. 1994;**344**(8922):563-570

[23] Park SJ, Park SW, Hong MK, Cheong SS, Lee CW, Kim JJ, et al. Stenting of unprotected left main coronary artery stenoses: Immediate and late outcomes. Journal of the American College of Cardiology. 1998;**31**(1):37-42

[24] Erglis A, Narbute I, Kumsars I, Jegere S, Mintale I, Zakke I, et al. A randomized comparison of paclitaxel-eluting stents versus bare-metal stents for treatment of unprotected left main coronary artery stenosis. Journal of the American College of Cardiology. 2007; **50**(6):491-497

[25] Mehilli J, Kastrati A, Byrne RA, Bruskina O, Iijima R, Schulz S, et al. Paclitaxel-versus sirolimus-eluting stents for unprotected left main coronary artery disease. Journal of the American College of Cardiology. 2009;**53**(19):1760-1768

[26] Buszman PE, Buszman PP, Banasiewicz-Szkróbka I, Milewski KP, Żurakowski A, Orlik B, et al. Left main stenting in comparison with surgical revascularization: 10-year outcomes of the (Left Main Coronary Artery Stenting)

LE MANS Trial. Cardiovascular Interventions. 2016;**9**(4):318-327

[27] Ong AT, Serruys PW, Mohr FW, Morice MC, Kappetein AP, Holmes DR Jr, et al. The SYNergy between percutaneous coronary intervention with TAXus and cardiac surgery (SYNTAX) study: Design, rationale, and run-in phase. American Heart Journal. 2006;**151**(6):1194-1204

[28] Boudriot E, Thiele H, Walther T, Liebetrau C, Boeckstegers P, Pohl T, et al. Randomized comparison of percutaneous coronary intervention with sirolimus-eluting stents versus coronary artery bypass grafting in unprotected left main stem stenosis. Journal of the American College of Cardiology. 2011;**57**(5):538-545

[29] Ahn JM, Roh JH, Kim YH, Park DW, Yun SC, Lee PH, et al. Randomized trial of stents versus bypass surgery for left main coronary artery disease: 5-year outcomes of the PRECOMBAT study. Journal of the American College of Cardiology. 2015; **65**(20):2198-2206

[30] Moynagh A, Salvatella N, Harb T, Darremont O, Boudou N, Dumonteil N, et al. Two-year outcomes of everolimus vs. paclitaxel-eluting stent for the treatment of unprotected left main lesions: A propensity score matching comparison of patients included in the French Left Main Taxus (FLM Taxus) and the LEft MAin Xience (LEMAX) registries. Eurointervention: Journal of Europcr in Collaboration with the Working Group on Interventional Cardiology of the European Society of Cardiology. 2013;**9**(4):452-462

[31] Cho Y, Shimura S, Aki A, Furuya H, Okada K, Ueda T. The SYNTAX score is correlated with long-term outcomes of coronary artery bypass grafting for complex coronary artery lesions. Interactive Cardiovascular and Thoracic Surgery. 2016;**23**(1):125-132

[32] Krishna N, Varma PK. Risk stratification in cardiac surgery. Indian Journal of Thoracic and Cardiovascular Surgery. 2015;**31**(3):224-233

[33] Chieffo A, Meliga E, Latib A, Park SJ, Onuma Y, Capranzano P, et al. Drug-eluting stent for left main coronary artery disease: The DELTA registry: A multicenter registry evaluating percutaneous coronary intervention versus coronary artery bypass grafting for left main treatment. JACC: Cardiovascular Interventions. 2012;**5**(7):718-727

[34] Park DW, Park SJ. Percutaneous coronary intervention of left main disease: Pre-and post-EXCEL (evaluation of XIENCE everolimus eluting stent versus coronary artery bypass surgery for effectiveness of left main revascularization) and NOBLE (Nordic-Baltic-British left main revascularization study) era. Circulation: Cardiovascular Interventions. 2017;**10**(6):e004792

[35] Sabatine MS, Bergmark BA, Murphy SA, O'Gara PT, Smith PK, Serruys PW, et al. Percutaneous coronary intervention with drug-eluting stents versus coronary artery bypass grafting in left main coronary artery disease: An individual patient data meta-analysis. The Lancet. 2021;**398**(10318): 2247-2257

[36] Gao L, Gao Z, Song Y, Guan C, Xu B, Chen J, et al. Long-term clinical outcomes of unprotected left main percutaneous coronary intervention: A large single-centre experience. Journal of Interventional Cardiology. 2021;**2021**:10. Article ID 8829686. DOI: 10.1155/2021/8829686

[37] Park DW, Seung KB, Kim YH, Lee JY, Kim WJ, Kang SJ, et al.

Long-term safety and efficacy of stenting versus coronary artery bypass grafting for unprotected left main coronary artery disease: 5-year results from the MAIN-COMPARE (Revascularization for Unprotected Left Main Coronary Artery Stenosis: Comparison of Percutaneous Coronary Angioplasty Versus Surgical Revascularization) registry. Journal of the American College of Cardiology. 2010; **56**(2):117-124

[38] Park DW, Ahn JM, Yun SC, Yoon YH, Kang DY, Lee PH, et al. 10-year outcomes of stents versus coronary artery bypass grafting for left main coronary artery disease. Journal of the American College of Cardiology. 2018;**72** (23 Part A):2813-2822

[39] Thuijs DJ, Kappetein AP, Serruys PW, Mohr FW, Morice MC, Mack MJ, et al. Percutaneous coronary intervention versus coronary artery bypass grafting in patients with three-vessel or left main coronary artery disease: 10-year follow-up of the multicentre randomised controlled SYNTAX trial. The Lancet. 2019; **394**(10206):1325-1334

[40] Park SJ, Kim YH. Percutaneous coronary intervention for unprotected left main coronary artery stenosis. Cardiology Clinics. 2010;**28**(1):81-95

[41] Hillis LD, Smith PK, Anderson JL, Bittl JA, Bridges CR, Byrne JG, et al. 2011 ACCF/AHA guideline for coronary artery bypass graft surgery: A report of the American College of Cardiology Foundation/American Heart Association Task Force on Practice Guidelines developed in collaboration with the American Association for Thoracic Surgery, Society of Cardiovascular Anesthesiologists, and Society of Thoracic Surgeons. Journal of the American College of Cardiology. 2011; **58**(24):e123-e210

[42] Lee DC, Oz MC, Weinberg AD, Ting W. Appropriate timing of surgical intervention after transmural acute myocardial infarction. The Journal of Thoracic and Cardiovascular Surgery. 2003;**125**(1):115-120

[43] Thielmann M, Neuhäuser M, Marr A, Herold U, Kamler M, Massoudy P, et al. Predictors and outcomes of coronary artery bypass grafting in ST elevation myocardial infarction. The Annals of thoracic surgery. 2007;**84**(1):17-24

[44] Steigen TK, Maeng M, Wiseth R, Erglis A, Kumsars I, Narbute I, et al. Randomized study on simple versus complex stenting of coronary artery bifurcation lesions: The Nordic bifurcation study. Circulation. 2006; **114**(18):1955-1961

[45] Hildick-Smith D, de Belder AJ, Cooter N, Curzen NP, Clayton TC, Oldroyd KG, et al. Randomized trial of simple versus complex drug-eluting stenting for bifurcation lesions: The British Bifurcation Coronary Study: Old, new, and evolving strategies. Circulation. 2010; **121**(10):1235-1243

[46] Ferenc M, Gick M, Comberg T, Rothe J, Valina C, Toma A, et al. Culotte stenting vs. TAP stenting for treatment of de-novo coronary bifurcation lesions with the need for side-branch stenting: The Bifurcations Bad Krozingen (BBK) II angiographic trial. European Heart J. 2016;**37**(45):3399-3405

[47] Colombo A, Bramucci E, Saccà S, Violini R, Lettieri C, Zanini R, et al. Randomized study of the crush technique versus provisional side-branch stenting in true coronary bifurcations: The CACTUS (Coronary Bifurcations: Application of the Crushing Technique Using Sirolimus-Eluting Stents) Study. Circulation. 2009;**119**(1):71-78

[48] Hildick-Smith D, Behan MW, Lassen JF, Chieffo A, Lefèvre T, Stankovic G, et al. The EBC TWO Study (European Bifurcation Coronary TWO) A Randomized Comparison of Provisional T-Stenting Versus a Systematic 2 Stent Culotte Strategy in Large Caliber True Bifurcations. Circulation: Cardiovascular Interventions. Sep 2016; **9**(9):e003643

[49] Chen SL. In the face of cunning enemy: DK crush writes legend. European Heart Journal. 2020;**41**:3763-3764

[50] Chen SL, Santoso T, Zhang JJ, Ye F, Xu YW, Fu Q, et al. A randomized clinical study comparing double kissing crush with provisional stenting for treatment of coronary bifurcation lesions: Results from the DKCRUSH-II (Double Kissing Crush versus Provisional Stenting Technique for Treatment of Coronary Bifurcation Lesions) trial. Journal of the American College of Cardiology. 2011; **57**(8):914-920

[51] Chen SL, Xu B, Han YL, Sheiban I, Zhang JJ, Ye F, et al. Clinical outcome after DK crush versus culotte stenting of distal left main bifurcation lesions: The 3-year follow-up results of the DKCRUSH-III study. Cardiovascular Interventions. 2015;**8**(10):1335-1342

[52] Chen SL, Zhang JJ, Han Y, Kan J, Chen L, Qiu C, et al. Double kissing crush versus provisional stenting for left main distal bifurcation lesions: DKCRUSH-V randomized trial. Journal of the American College of Cardiology. 2017;**70**(21):2605-2617

[53] Hildick-Smith D, Egred M, Banning A, Brunel P, Ferenc M, Hovasse T, et al. The European bifurcation club Left Main Coronary Stent study: A randomized comparison of stepwise provisional vs. systematic dual stenting strategies (EBC MAIN). European Heart Journal. 2021;**42**(37): 3829-3839

[54] Kang SJ, Ahn JM, Song H, Kim WJ, Lee JY, Park DW, et al. Comprehensive intravascular ultrasound assessment of stent area and its impact on restenosis and adverse cardiac events in 403 patients with unprotected left main disease. Circulation: Cardiovascular Interventions. 2011;**4**(6):562-569

[55] Stone GW, Witzenbichler B, Weisz G, Rinaldi MJ, Neumann FJ, Metzger DC, et al. Platelet reactivity and clinical outcomes after coronary artery implantation of drug-eluting stents (ADAPT-DES): A prospective multicentre registry study. The Lancet. 2013;**382**(9892):614-623

[56] Gao XF, Ge Z, Kong XQ, Kan J, Han L, Lu S, et al. 3-year outcomes of the ULTIMATE trial comparing intravascular ultrasound versus angiography-guided drug-eluting stent implantation. Cardiovascular Interventions. 2021;**14**(3):247-257

[57] Farkouh ME, Domanski M, Dangas GD, Godoy LC, Mack MJ, Siami FS, et al. Long-term survival following multivessel revascularization in patients with diabetes: The FREEDOM follow-on study. Journal of the American College of Cardiology. 2019;**73**(6): 629-638

[58] Cho SC, Park DW, Park SJ. Percutaneous coronary intervention and coronary artery bypass grafting for the treatment of left main coronary artery disease. Korean Circulation Journal. 2019;**49**(5):369-383

[59] Dehnee A, Gerula C, Mazza V, Maher J, Dhruvakumar S, Kaluski E. The functional SYNTAX score: A huge step forward or research in motion? Journal of Invasive Cardiology. 2012;**24**(6): 304-305